Diet for Life

DIET FOR LIFE

A Metabolism Expert's Commonsense Plan for Overcoming Obesity

By David S. H. Bell, MB, FACE

As told to Anita Smith

Forewords by James H. O'Keefe, MD, FACE and Ralph A. DeFronzo, MD, FACE

Court Street Press

Montgomery | Louisville

Court Street Presss
P.O. Box 1588
Montgomery, AL 36102

Published in the United States by Court Street Press, a division of NewSouth, Inc., Montgomery, Alabama.

Library of Congress Cataloging-in-Publication Data

Bell, David. S. H.
Diet for life : a metabolism expert's commonsense plan for overcoming obesity / by David S. H. Bell as told to Anita Smith; forewords by James H. O'Keefe and Ralph A. DeFronzo.
p. cm.
Includes index.
ISBN-13: 978-1-58838-224-5
ISBN-10: 1-58838-224-9
1. Bell, David. S. H.—Health. 2. Overweight persons—Biography. 3. Endocrinologists—Biography. 4. Weight loss. 5. Obesity. I. Smith, Anita. II. Title.
RC628.B356 2008
362.196'3980092—dc22
[B]

2007051311

Design by Randall Williams
Printed in the United States of America
by the Maple-Vail Book Manufacturing Group

IN MEMORY OF MY MOTHER,

VIOLET BELL

(1919–2007)

Contents

Foreword

"You Only Have One Life"

James H. O'Keefe, MD, FACE

In *Diet for Life*, Dr. David Bell, one of America's foremost experts in diabetes, metabolism, and cardiovascular disease, shares his personal story about how he has permanently lost one hundred pounds of excess weight and restored his health. Dr. Bell was able to do this by using a rather unconventional approach, consuming only one meal a day. The other component of Dr. Bell's One-Plus-One Weight-Loss Plan is an hour of exercise daily. These two fundamental action steps of the "Diet for Life" program—consuming fewer calories and burning more calories—lie at the heart of any successful long-term strategy for achieving and maintaining ideal weight.

If your goal is to live a longer and healthier life, the single most powerful dietary change you can make is simply to reduce your overall calorie intake. In animals, including primates, cutting calorie intake by about one-third markedly improves longevity and vigor. Studies to date in humans indicate that calorie restriction reduces inflammation immediately and improves most of the common chronic diseases including high blood pressure, diabetes, and high cholesterol.

The ideal way to cut calories is to avoid eating, especially the calorie-dense processed fare that is ubiquitous in our modern world. A common dietary strategy is to consume five or six small meals throughout the day. My dietitian wife, Joan O'Keefe, finds that most people who try to do this end up overeating, and are unable to achieve or maintain successful weight loss. On the other hand, when you eat only one meal a day (in effect, fast throughout the day), you are limited in the amount of calories you can consume in one setting, particularly if you stick to whole natural foods like fresh produce, fresh meat, fish, nuts, berries, etc.

ALTHOUGH MODERN HUMANS have evolved rapidly from the technological and social aspects, genetically we are evolving at a glacial pace. Genetic experts tell us that our human genome has changed minimally since our ancient ancestors walked out of their caves ten thousand years ago. We are designed by nature to thrive best when we eat like the hunter-gatherer that our DNA says we still are. Those hunter-gatherers spent much of their day walking, carrying, climbing, and running to procure their food. At the end of the day they pooled their collected produce and game and had their one large meal.

America today—and much of the western world—is a land that indulges our freedom of choice. You can choose to have green hair and blue eyes, or to watch Sponge Bob Square Pants around the clock, or for your morning coffee, you can choose to have a vanilla, half-caf, 1 percent, extra-hot, no-foam latte—but you can't yet choose your genes. Those genes, the blueprint to build and maintain you, specify the kinds of foods upon which you will either thrive or decay.

That's why not all diets are created equal, and why food cannot be like fashion fads that come and go.

Dr. Bell's "Diet for Life" works so well for achieving ideal weight and restoring vigorous health because it prescribes the eating and exercise patterns for which we remain genetically designed. Why does a cactus thrive in the Arizona desert and not in the rain forest near Seattle? For the same reason that we thrive best when we eat whole natural foods in modest quantities and make time for exercise each day—nature made us this way.

AS RANDY GLASBERGEN quipped in one of his cartoons: "What fits into your busy schedule better, exercising one hour a day or being dead 24 hours a day?" If we had a pill that replicated all of the benefits conferred by daily vigorous exercise, we doctors would be out of business. Most Americans

---

JAMES H. O'KEEFE, MD, is a clinical cardiologist, medical school professor, researcher, and author based in Kansas City, Missouri. Among his books is *The Forever Young Diet & Lifestyle*, co-written with his registered-dietitian wife, Joan.

need to exercise every day—exercise has the power to revolutionize our health and vitality like nothing else can. Studies consistently show that if your goal is to achieve and maintain an ideal body weight, you will need to exercise for 45 minutes to 90 minutes daily. You can break the exertion up into two sessions, just as long as the total daily time spent exercising adds up to about one hour.

Many of us who exercise do so first thing in the morning, even though it means we have to roll out of bed a bit earlier. I notice that I feel generally better during the day if I have exercised that morning. I find that an early morning workout is the only way I can predictably get my exercise done every day, and working out first thing in the morning assures that you will get your fitness activity done before the rest of the world wakes up and has a chance to start harassing you with obligations. As an added perk, you won't have that nagging guilt about getting your exercise hanging over your head for the rest of the day. If you wait till after work, many people feel too tired, hungry, or emotionally exhausted to muster the energy it takes to overcome their inertia.

My wife Joan doesn't allow herself the luxury of her morning shower until her exercise is done.

What if you can't seem to drag yourself out of bed in the morning to exercise, and you find you're too tired to get it done after work? A refreshing exercise session over the lunch hour may just be your ticket to fitness. Get out for a brisk 30-minute walk over the noon hour instead of bogging yourself down with a load of calories that leave you with post-lunch fatigue and sluggishness. Exercise in the middle of the day is not just convenient but also invigorating.

Studies show that a 30- to 60-minute workout at lunchtime lowers stress, improves productivity, and leaves you happier for the rest of the day. I personally find this to be my favorite time to exercise, and I do it whenever I get the chance. I like to think of life as a grand adventure that I need to train for so I can fully appreciate all of its beauty and opportunity.

Follow Dr. Bell's "Diet for Life" and you will get back down to your ideal weight and thrive with vigor. You only have one life, make it the best it can be.

Foreword

"Energy In = Energy Out"

Ralph A. DeFronzo, MD, FACE

Over the last two decades, obesity has reached epidemic proportions in westernized countries. In the United States 66 percent of adults (133.6 million) are frankly obese or overweight. Most alarming, 4.7 percent of adults (nine million) are considered to be morbidly obese. Despite the well-established causal associations between obesity versus Type 2 diabetes, metabolic syndrome, hypertension, coronary artery disease, stroke, gall bladder disease, cancer, arthritis, and many other serious medical problems, the majority of adults find it difficult to maintain their body weight within the normal range, especially with advancing age. Even more disturbing is the rising incidence (17 percent) of childhood obesity with the development of diseases, e.g., Type 2 diabetes, previously considered to begin in adulthood.

The key to understanding the maintenance of normal weight is embodied in the energy balance equation: ENERGY IN = ENERGY OUT. Simply stated, if energy (food) intake is excessive or if physical activity is insufficient, weight gain will occur.

Many myths have been generated about the thermogenic benefit of one food type over another. The truth remains that a calorie is a calorie is a calorie, whether the calorie comes from carbohydrate, fat, or protein. Therefore, it is essential that the total number of calories consumed not exceed the amount of energy expended, and that the distribution of calories be balanced with regard to carbohydrate, fat, and protein.

In this book, Dr. Bell espouses the one-meal-per-day weight-loss program, which allowed him to lose more than one hundred pounds and maintain this weight loss over a period of more than four years. This one-meal-per-day dietary plan, that I have followed since age 18, has maintained my body weight within the normal range for over 45 years.

Most individuals who maintain ideal body weight employ some form of "controlled eating" plan, i.e., they have a certain body image and they regulate their appetite to achieve/maintain that body image. For Dr. Bell and myself, we have found the one-meal-per-day plan easy to implement and simple to follow.

When switching from the more usual two to three meals per day to one meal per day, individuals will feel hungry during the day but this sensation of hunger usually subsides within the first week. It is important that individuals maintain an active work schedule, and avoid food cues, especially during this initial transition period. As pointed out by Dr. Bell, the one-meal-per-day approach may not fit all individuals. Therefore, it is essential that whatever dietary program that is adopted be one that the person can follow.

THE SECOND PART of the One-Plus-One Weight-Loss Plan is exercise, which has two benefits. First, and most importantly, it improves cardiovascular fitness and reduces the likelihood of experiencing a heart attack or stroke. Second, it burns calories and assists in promoting weight loss. However, most individuals fail to appreciate the magnitude of the energy deficit that can be created by mild- to moderate-intensity exercise. Thus, if one walks (or jogs lightly) one mile in 15 minutes, the number of calories expended is 90 to 100.

Maintenance of this pace for one hour will result in a total expenditure of about 400 calories. If one combines one hour a day of mild or moderate exercise with a decrease in food (caloric) intake of six hundred calories a day, this will provide a weight loss of one pound every 3.5 days (3500 calories = one pound) or two pounds per week.

Most individuals who enter structured weight loss programs are success-

---

RALPH A. DEFRONZO, MD, is Professor of Medicine, Director of Diabetes, University of Texas Health Science Center in San Antonio. He is widely known for his research work in obesity and the body's resistance to insulin.

ful while they are in the program. However, once the structured program ends, weight regain is the norm.

Both Dr. Bell and I have found the One-Plus-One Weight Loss/Maintenance Plan to be highly successful for ourselves personally and for our patients.

Try it! You'll like it!

Prologue

My Dangerous Moment of Truth

My life began anew at a health convention in June 2003 in New Orleans, Louisiana. At the time, I was a 59-year-old fat physician specializing in diabetes, metabolism and endocrinology. To this day, I'm still amazed that while I was in New Orleans or shortly afterward I didn't become a 59-year-old fat, dead physician.

Standing 6 feet 5 inches tall, I can carry a bit more weight than the average person. But not three hundred pounds plus a few! I had been fat most of my life, dating back to my childhood. Through the years, eating what I wanted was important to me. It was more important than getting rid of an ugly gut. It was more important than following the health advice I gave my patients, many of whom had diabetes. If the truth were known, my basic attitude was that diets and drugs were for patients; they weren't for me. I was the doctor. I always thought I was perfectly healthy, that I would live forever or close to it. In fact, I really thought I was not at all vulnerable, about as close to invincible as one can hope for.

Up until that point in 2003 it seemed to me I had gotten by with my way of doing things. But time was marching on. I wasn't as young as I used to be. And I was continuing to maintain a pressure-packed academic-medicine schedule of seeing patients, conducting research, writing scientific papers, and traveling frequently to make clinical presentations. Even though I appeared healthy, my wife of more than 30 years, Jocelyn, had really been on my case about getting a physical.

Typical of my stubborn, independent way of doing things, I had made no move to get a physical. However, while attending the American Diabetes Association meeting in New Orleans, I decided to pacify Jocelyn by at least getting a couple of free health screenings. Those screenings were easily accessible to convention-goers in locations scattered throughout the Exhibit Hall where drug companies and other vendors had their booths.

As I paid a visit to the exhibits during a break between convention sessions, I thought, "Since I have a bit of time before my next meeting here, I'll just get a cholesterol test done." I got the cholesterol test, and I was favorably impressed with the result. It wasn't a bad cholesterol reading at all—particularly for a 300-pound man.

So, with the acceptable cholesterol result in hand, I decided that I had enough time to venture confidently a step further and get my blood pressure checked. In the Exhibit Hall I found a state-of-the-art machine that measured not only the blood pressure but also the resistance of the arteries. The machine was set in motion, and I waited for it to display my blood pressure reading. In the seconds I waited, I felt no anxiety, no worry at all about what the test might show. For me this was just routine. My mind already was on that next meeting I would be attending at the convention, and, always very important to me, where we were going to eat that night.

The two numbers for my blood pressure reading flashed in front of me. I sat there looking at the top number that reflected my "systolic pressure"—the pressure of my blood against the walls of my arteries while my heart was busy contracting to pump blood. And I sat there looking at the bottom number that reflected my "diastolic pressure"—the pressure of my blood against the artery walls when my heart was at rest, between heartbeats.

I was totally stunned by the reading I saw! The numbers that appeared before my eyes were not anything with which I could connect, nothing I could relate to myself. This blood pressure reading at which I now gazed in that Exhibit Hall was light years removed from any reading I could associate with me. From my view, these numbers certainly could have nothing to do with David Bell.

I mean, in my years of practicing medicine, I had seen blood pressure readings like that. I had seen them in some of my own patients. Whenever I saw such a reading, I sprang into action immediately to minister to the patient. For I well knew that a patient with a blood pressure reading like that was in jeopardy, in effect sitting on a time bomb in his body ready to explode. I knew the patient needed all the medical help I and my colleagues could give—help we could give as rapidly as possible that day, not that week or month. I also knew bringing a dangerous blood pressure reading like that under control required a great deal of cooperation from the patient himself.

On that memorable summer day in 2003, as I stared at the blood pressure reading in an Exhibit Hall in New Orleans, I wasn't looking at someone else's blood pressure reading. I was looking at my own.

The reading was a startling 190 over 110. (Anything above 140 over 90 is reason for concern, and ideally the reading should be 120 over 80 or less.) When I saw that 190/110 reading, my first response was to become impatient because I felt this blood pressure machine had a problem. I thought, "This machine is useless!! This machine can't be accurate. This is just not true."

At that point I was due at a board meeting being held in conjunction with the convention—a meeting of a medical-journal editorial board on which I served. As I made my way to my meeting, I struggled unsuccessfully to push that blood pressure reading into the back of my mind.

As soon as my meeting was over, I rushed back to the Exhibit Hall and back to that same blood pressure machine. My plan was that I would give this aggravating machine another chance to get the reading right. So I went about the process of letting the machine re-check my blood pressure. In my mind, the machine had had a little time to settle down and this re-check would produce a normal-range blood pressure reading, which of course would be accurate for me. But this "happy-ending scenario" I had envisioned was not to be. This time my blood pressure reading was even higher. It was 210 over 120—alarming, stroke level blood pressure.

Still I could not accept this. I continued to believe that the machine was really inaccurate. I thought, "I have to find a qualified human being to take my blood pressure." So I quickly walked to a nearby first aid station in the Exhibit Hall and asked a nurse there to take it for me. She graciously obliged, and proceeded to put the cuff on my arm to get a manual reading. When she looked up at me and announced the results, I didn't like what I heard. She said, "It's 195 over 120." Then she took it again; same reading.

She took it again; same reading.

Truth was being pounded into my brain. My time for denial officially had come to an end. The problem at hand was not a faulty blood pressure machine. The problem certainly wasn't a nurse who didn't know how to take blood pressure. The problem was that I had a problem, a serious one.

I was very concerned. No, I was more than concerned. I was flat scared. I thought I could have a stroke at any minute. In fact, I knew that if a person has raging blood pressure at that level, that person is a sitting duck for a stroke. Even though I was feeling no symptoms such as dizziness or headache, I knew I *still* was a sitting duck.

In medical circles, high blood pressure generally is referred to as "hypertension." However, regardless of whether one refers to the condition as "high blood pressure" or "hypertension," it also has the well-deserved nickname of being "the silent killer." That's because this stealthy condition often is very silent as it sets the stage for disaster to occur inside the human body. A lot of people who have high blood pressure have no symptoms to sound a warning to them—at least no symptoms that they notice. As I stood there in that New Orleans convention center, I realized to my great shock that I now was one of those people.

My mind began to race. Over and over, the same simple thought kept going through my mind, "Hey, this is *very* dangerously high blood pressure." I knew I needed to take action right away. I couldn't just wander around this convention, going to meetings and looking at exhibits, as if nothing was wrong.

I pondered whether I should return home right then to Birmingham, Alabama. I thought, "Do I get a taxi to the airport immediately and take a Southwest Airlines plane back to Birmingham and admit myself to the hospital and get some of my physician colleagues to minister to me?" I decided no, that was not the route I would take. If I did that, they likely would only keep me in the hospital overnight and send me home, in the meantime filling me with all these intravenous drugs that would give me a headache that would last three days. Again, in typical fashion, I decided to handle it myself.

The first thing I knew I had to do was to get hold of some medicine to bring this blood pressure under control. I was so intent on getting the medicine that I didn't take time at the crowded convention center to hail a taxi. Walking would be quicker, I thought. Since I was in downtown New Orleans, logic told me that I wouldn't have to walk far before I found a drugstore. Wrong! I struck out walking in search of a drugstore—in that sweltering humid heat for which New Orleans is so known in the summer months. I walked a block in search of a drugstore. I walked another block, and another block, and another. (Get this picture: A physician who is in medical jeopardy, out on a city sidewalk alone, doing all this walking and huffing and puffing, in the heat, under stress, with the full knowledge he has out-of-control blood pressure. Now, go figure this logic!)

I walked five blocks before I finally found a drugstore. By the time I found one, I was really huffing and puffing and perspiring profusely. But still my quest was not over. When I walked into the drugstore and asked for the pharmacy, much to my surprise I was told that this particular drugstore didn't have a pharmacy! (I didn't know they had drugstores that didn't have pharmacies. Why would they call them "drugstores" if they don't sell drugs . . . ???)

Again I took off on foot. This time I walked another three blocks and hit paydirt. I found a drugstore that had a pharmacy. I got some medication for high blood pressure. Needless to say, I began taking the pills immediately.

As the medication took hold in my body, gradually my blood pressure readings began to ease downward in the hours and days that followed.

But I knew no medication on the face of the earth would be enough to dig me out of this deep, dangerous hole I had gotten myself into. In addition to taking the medication, I knew I had to do at least three things that added up to the biggest changes I had ever made in my life.

First of all, I had to confront who and what I was. I was a fat child who had become a fat adult—a fat, very unhealthy adult.

Secondly, I had to commit myself to the goal of becoming a healthy man.

Thirdly, in order to become a healthy man and maintain a healthy lifestyle, I had to do what to me had been unthinkable for years. I had to devise and carry out a diet-and-exercise plan to lose a considerable amount of weight and keep it off, and to get in shape and stay in shape.

Thus, at age 59, when my life easily could have ended or have been severely limited by a stroke or heart attack, I had a chance to embark on a new life.

Today, almost five years later, I'm lean and fit, at least a hundred pounds slimmer and keeping it off—and enjoying normal blood pressure. Getting to this satisfying point in life hasn't been as tough a journey as I thought it would be. In fact, I've had some fun with the journey, and I continue to have fun with it. The life I have today is a life I want to shout about. It's a life I'd like to see many others enjoy. That's why I wrote this book.

Part I

Taking Action

Chapter 1

"What's Up, Doc?"

In the months following the scary experience I had in New Orleans, I began dropping weight steadily and quite noticeably.

Those who knew me had never before seen me lose weight like that. As one might expect, people began asking me about my weight loss. One setting in which I received a steady stream of questions was in my office, where I maintained a busy schedule seeing patients. My patients were asking a lot of questions. They were extremely curious. In some cases, my patients were not only curious; they also were *concerned.* They were worried about me.

Needless to say, the issue of weight had come up many times in my office—mostly the issue of *my patients' weight.* There were occasions when I felt it prudent to urge overweight patients to bring their weight under control. Since I was treating many patients suffering from diabetes, weight management was an important part of managing their care.

Whenever I had talked about weight with patients, my own overweight condition of course was quite obvious. As I spoke about the health-related hazards of carrying too much weight, I sat behind my desk with my gut spilling over onto the desk, or I stood in an examining room with my bulky form visibly protruding under my white jacket.

Even though I advised my patients about weight management, I certainly was not the pushiest of doctors on the subject of weight. I didn't tend to harp on it. The reason didn't have to do with my being self-conscious about lecturing to others while having a weight problem of my own. Instead, the reason had to do with my pessimism about patients being successful in reversing their weight problems.

Over the years I had observed that no matter how pushy or even downright "ugly" a doctor gets with patients about weight loss, people don't lose weight and keep it off. That's particularly true in this plentiful United States where food is so available and where eating—or I should say *overeating*—is so important to people. I was well aware that with most of my patients it was an exercise in futility to expect them to lose weight and keep it off. Many studies show that even when people go on weight-loss programs and succeed in losing weight that, within two years, more than 90 percent are back to weighing as much as they did before they started their weight-loss programs, and in all too many cases they weigh even *more*.

An Overweight Doctor Draws Teasing from Patients

I had many patients whom I had treated for quite a number of years. My patients and I felt comfortable with one another. It wasn't unusual for my patients to joke with me and not unusual for me to joke with them. I've always been friendly with my patients. It has never been a part of my professional makeup to be "stand-offish" with patients or to want them to be overly formal with me. I certainly didn't want them to fear me.

So it wasn't unusual for a patient to come out with a chiding comment now and then about *my* weight—especially when I was talking to that patient about his or her weight.

I have walked into an examination room and heard a patient say something to the effect of, "You're not getting any smaller, Doc, are you?"

I've been in a number of conversations with an overweight patient who had diabetes, and had the conversation go something like this: I would say, "Now, you really need to get some of your weight off." And the patient would say, "Doc, you're really one to talk!" To which I would grin and reply, "Me doctor. You patient. Drugs and diets are for patients. And, you have diabetes; I don't!"

The sad thing is that I was not totally teasing in such conversations. Until I saw my skyrocketing blood pressure reading in New Orleans in June 2003, I think I really deep down did believe that diets and drugs were for my patients but not for me. I'm convinced I held the opinion that I could just keep on eating what I wanted and weighing whatever and that nothing bad was going to happen to me.

A Skinnier Doctor Draws Concern from Patients

Just as I had received comments from my patients when I was their fat doctor, I received many questions from my patients as I began to drop pounds following my "moment of truth" in New Orleans.

The questions didn't come as a surprise to me. In fact, I would have been surprised if there had not been questions. I mean, I had been overweight all the years these patients had known me. Now all of a sudden there was a drastic change in my weight. Instead of my being a few pounds heavier each time a patient saw me, I was considerably slimmer each time.

I had given some thought as to what I would tell my patients when they asked about my weight loss. For a while, I was going to answer their questions with a general rather than a specific answer. The reason was that I did not want to reveal the details of my rather creative weight-loss program until I had a chance to see if it really worked.

In my mind, my weight-loss program would not really work until I could both (a) *lose the weight,* and (b) for a sustained period—let's say a year—prove to myself that I could *keep the weight off.*

So, when my patients started asking, "Doc, how are you losing all this weight?" I responded with a "broad-brush" but nevertheless truthful answer: "Diet and exercise."

Predictably, that answer fell short in satisfying the curiosity of many of my patients. So, with those patients I knew well and with whom I felt especially comfortable, I added some joking banter. This was a typical exchange in this little comedy routine:

A patient would come in, often concerned about my weight loss, and say, "Doc, are you okay?"

"Yeah."

"You don't have cancer or anything, do you?"

"No."

"You haven't been sick? You haven't been ill?"

"No, not as far as I know."

"You've lost a lot of weight."

"Yeah, I know. I've been trying."

"How are you doing it?"

"Diet and exercise."

"But Doc, you're really dropping a *lot* of weight. Like, specifically, what are you doing?"

"Well, if I tell you, you won't tell anyone else, right?"

"Right. I won't tell."

"Okay. Well, I have sex three times a day and I'm too *tired* to eat."

Now, I realize that might sound a bit risqué to some who are reading this book. But, as I told you, I was a friend to my patients. I had been with a number of these patients through some pretty rough health crises in their lives.

I never made that comment without getting laughter from the patient—be it a man or a woman. Once I made the comment, they all tended to look at me quizzically for a millisecond, and then laugh, and then come forth with their varied responses.

From a couple of my female patients, I got this ladylike response, "Well my *husband* would like that!" To which I replied, "Well, why wouldn't *you* like it? Why just your *husband?*"

From a quick-witted man whom I had treated for years I got a raucous laugh and then this prompt response, "Doc, lying will get you to hell just as quick as stealing!"

Chapter 2

My Weight-Loss Plan

The program I used to lose weight in late 2003 and on into 2004—*and* the program I have used to keep the weight off since then—is an unusual regimen. It is a plan I devised for myself. It is a plan that has worked for me. It is a plan that I have in fact come to enjoy. In my view, it also is a plan that would work for a lot of other people—not everyone, but a lot of people.

I've christened the plan "Diet for Life, the One-Plus-One Weight-Loss Plan." The name implies what the program is all about. The last part of the name simply means eating one meal a day and doing one hour of exercise per day. And the first part of the name implies that this is one diet plan that you can live with for the rest of your life.

I came up with this regimen because it fits me and my lifestyle. I came up with it also because, in my opinion, it makes sense as a healthy, effective way to lose weight and to keep it off.

This is my journey in coming up with the One-Plus-One Plan and putting it into action:

Big Decision Time

Let's go back to where it all started, with my stroke-level blood pressure reading while I was attending the meeting in New Orleans.

For me, at that point it was crunch-time in my life, time for a decision. We all come face-to-face with those big decisions in our lives—those decisions in which we balance one set of factors against another set of factors and decide whether to make a major change.

Most of us don't have to think very long before we recall one of these major decision-making periods in our lives.

Like deciding whether to try to accomplish certain career goals in a current work situation, or instead to take a chance and accept a very new and different job.

Or deciding whether to make a long-term commitment to an individual who is a romantic interest, or instead risk the possibility that, without a commitment, that person could go in another direction and leave you all alone.

Or deciding whether to leave the comfort and familiarity of living in one place, or instead start a new life in another locale far away from longtime surroundings and family and friends.

Remember that the decision I faced in 2003 related to my health and well-being. In my mind, that type of decision ranks pretty high in importance on the totem pole. *As I saw the decision I faced in 2003, it was a choice between two options:*

Option One: Try to control my blood pressure with medication alone, and continue on with eating too much and exercising too little.

Option Two: Make a commitment to give up my old bad habits related to diet and exercise, and embark on a stricter and healthier diet and exercise regimen to bring about a substantial weight loss.

In New Orleans, I set my sights on Option Two. In the first few days after I left New Orleans, I would have reason to reinforce that this was the only decision I could make.

Putting on the Brakes

Once I realized my situation in New Orleans, I immediately began cutting down drastically on my food intake. Too, I immediately stopped drinking any kind of alcohol. (Alcoholic beverages add calories. Also, alcohol itself can make your blood pressure climb.)

Even with eating less, drinking none, and taking those blood pressure pills religiously, my stubborn blood pressure took its own sweet time in coming down to acceptable levels.

It was on a Monday when I made that stunning discovery about my frighteningly high blood pressure. Even putting into play my decades of experience in treating hypertensive patients with medication, there was no "instant magic" to bringing my own blood pressure under control.

In New Orleans, after I *finally* located that drugstore with a pharmacy in downtown New Orleans, I purchased two different medications to control hypertension. I was familiar with the use of both medications and knew them to be highly effective.

Even with taking both medications, my blood pressure readings did not go down very much in the first critical hours. So I added a *third* blood pressure control medication. Still my blood pressure reading remained extremely high Tuesday, Wednesday, Thursday, and Friday.

All during that week, I was still "on the road." When I left the meeting in New Orleans, I headed out on a lecture trip first to South Carolina and then to Pennsylvania before coming home that weekend. I had made prior commitments to make clinical presentations to some groups of physicians, and I felt I should not cancel those speaking engagements. Looking back, I question the wisdom of my decision to continue on that lecture trip in light of my blood pressure situation. I'm a lucky man, for I suffered no major health crisis on the trip. If I were to face a similar situation again, I hope I would be prudent enough to return sooner to familiar home and healthcare surroundings.

Everywhere I went on that lecture trip, I had my blood pressure taken. When I had my blood pressure checked on Saturday morning and it still was quite high a full five days after I had discovered my condition, I'll have to admit my level of concern was high. But then, around noon Saturday, I saw a breakthrough in the right direction.

It was almost like a high fever suddenly breaking and coming down substantially. My blood pressure had reached acceptable levels. Still, that "acceptable level" was on the upper end of normal. I knew I had a ways to go to attain ideal blood pressure readings. And I realized I had to work at keeping those readings at normal levels.

Not Just a Temporary Situation

Out of all this stress came a dawning of reality for me. It made an impression on me that my blood pressure had reached the heights it had without my even having noticeable symptoms, and that it had required five days after my "moment of truth" in New Orleans to bring the situation under control. What I was dealing with was not a "passing condition." It was a condition I would have to manage and monitor the rest of my life.

Being a physician, I have known since early in my medical training that one's chances of getting a little high blood pressure increase with age. If you reach age 55 and you're not hypertensive, there's a 90 percent chance that before you die you will be hypertensive to some degree. And that's even if you are not severely overweight. (If you *are* severely overweight, you're *really* at high risk for having high blood pressure.)

Since I was 59 years of age, I knew I certainly qualified for being in the "getting older" category. However, in June 2003 I was under no delusions that I had "mild hypertension," and I was under no delusions that I could attribute my situation solely to the aging process. What I had was more like what we doctors call "malignant hypertension"—a very dangerous situation. And, any way I cut it, I knew that my high blood pressure was tied in with my being severely overweight.

Blood Pressure Pills Not Enough

In my view, making a decision back in 2003 to lose a substantial amount of weight was, as the younger folks say these days, a "no-brainer." Based on my knowledge as a physician, I realized in spades in June 2003 that I indeed was a lucky man to have learned I had a life-threatening health problem before that problem blindsided me with death or disability.

Too, also from my realistic view as a physician, I knew I was by no means out of the woods just by finding a drugstore and getting some blood pressure pills.

If you're as overweight as I was (or even close), pulling that weight down is an essential ingredient in the recipe to control high blood pressure, or hypertension. It's a simple correlation: The *bad news* is that if you are decidedly overweight *and* hypertensive and you remain overweight and perhaps gain even more weight, the hypertension will stay high and likely go even higher. The *good news* is that if you're hypertensive and you lose weight, the hypertension tends to go down.

Judging by what I had learned in my medical training and had seen in my medical practice, a sky-high blood pressure like I had was going to require *both* pills and weight loss to bring the hypertension under control and keep it under control. I knew, too, that I had to take the weight-loss journey not only to combat my high blood pressure, but also to ward off a number of other health problems that are associated with being overweight. (*Note:* I will discuss the myriad of overweight-related health problems later in this Book.)

The bottom line was that I had to get off a lot of the weight I was carrying and keep it off. Never in my life had I both (1) lost weight and (2) really kept the weight off after I lost it. The time had come for action.

Starting with the Basics

For a number of years, my medical career had included an increasing number of speaking engagements and participation in national and international committees. This meant considerable travel. It meant mingling with physicians from all over the world—many of whom were, like myself, specialists in metabolism.

Thus, wherever I had gone, the subject of weight-loss plans had come up often. Weight-loss plans had been (and still are) a frequent subject among physicians with whom I interact.

As I've said, until 2003 I didn't connect these weight-loss plans with myself. I connected them mostly with my patients. Nevertheless, I was quite familiar with the basic tenets of a good weight-loss plan.

One of these basic tenets is that there is a difference between a "diet plan" and a good "weight-loss" plan. To have a good weight-loss plan, it's not enough to restrict calories in controlled dieting. You also need to add the second component—exercise. So I knew that whatever I did was going to be a combination of diet and exercise.

Another facet I had learned through the years that stuck with me was that there are "three beginning steps" you must take when you're embarking on a good weight-loss program:

The Three Beginning Steps

As I sat on the airplane en route to my home in Birmingham, Alabama, more than a week after my episode in New Orleans, I gave some thought to how those Three Beginning Steps applied to me as I embarked on a weight-loss program:

◊ **Step Number One: Get yourself on some reliable scales and weigh.** It makes sense to me when weight-loss experts say it's important for people to weigh. I had heard for many years that people who tend to keep their weight under control tend to be obsessive/compulsive scale users. I knew that if someone is starting a weight-loss program—as was the case with me in 2003—it was very important to get on the scales at the beginning of the program and then continue to weigh often. I understood the logic of all this. I mean, you have to know where you are with most anything in order to know where you're going. The way I look at it, there's nothing that will convince you more that you're really fat than looking down at the scales and seeing a dreaded number that tells you that you are fat! However, I will admit to you that I was not looking forward to Step Number One. I was not looking forward to stepping on those scales.

◊ **Step Number Two: Find a healthy diet that you can use as a part of your weight-loss program.** Find a diet that fits you. Find a diet that will be effective in controlling your calorie intake. And find a diet that is a healthy one. I knew that to lose the considerable amount of weight I wanted to lose I needed to find a healthy diet that was around 1,800 calories a day. Even as I sat on that airplane going home on that June 2003 weekend, I had some ideas in mind for a rather unusual diet for myself.

◊ **Step Number Three: Identify an effective, healthy exercise regimen that you can use as a part of your weight-loss program.** As I thought about exercise, I focused on my own challenge with an exercise program: I had to commit myself to be faithful and consistent with exercising. Up until that point, I had "dabbled" with exercise—a little here, a little there, but not enough exercise and not consistent exercise. I knew that I needed to identify an effective exercise program I would use for one hour every day.

A Sunday Morning Surprise

It had been a long time since I had enough courage to step on some reliable scales and weigh. I had been in tune with reality enough to know that most conventional scales would not even register my weight. The reason is that most conventional scales will not register a weight above 300 pounds. (And I qualified!) The weight limit on the scales I used for patients in my own office was 300 pounds. Many home bathroom scales, including those at our home, won't register a weight above 280 pounds.

If someone had asked me to guess my weight at the time I experienced that "moment of truth" in New Orleans, my guess would have been "perhaps as much as 310." (Although I certainly would not have shared my "guess" with anyone!)

Now, if you're tall—which I am—that can give you an edge to carry a little more weight than your shorter friends. However, no matter how tall you are, there's still a limit to how much you should weigh. Even though I am 6 feet, 5 inches tall, I knew that even my tall frame should be carrying around considerably less weight than it was carrying.

So, even going by my guess that I weighed around 310 pounds when I learned about my sky-rocketing blood pressure in June 2003, at that weight I was clearly about 100 pounds overweight!

By the time I got around to actually stepping on the scales and weighing, it had been almost two weeks since my New Orleans "awakening." During that time, I knew I had dropped quite a few pounds. In the days following my "New Orleans moment of truth," I ate very, very little—actually, practically nothing. And I could feel that my clothes were becoming considerably looser. I figure that during that almost-two-week period, I lost at least 7 or 8 pounds, perhaps as much as 10 to 12 pounds.

So, when I decided to step on the scales—after I arrived home from my New Orleans meeting and the lecture trip—I really thought I might be under 300 pounds.

Just to be on the safe side with that 300-pound limit for most scales, I decided to weigh on a pair of professional medical-clinic scales that were designed to weigh obese people—including people who weighed more than 300 pounds. The scales I had in mind were in the Geriatric Department

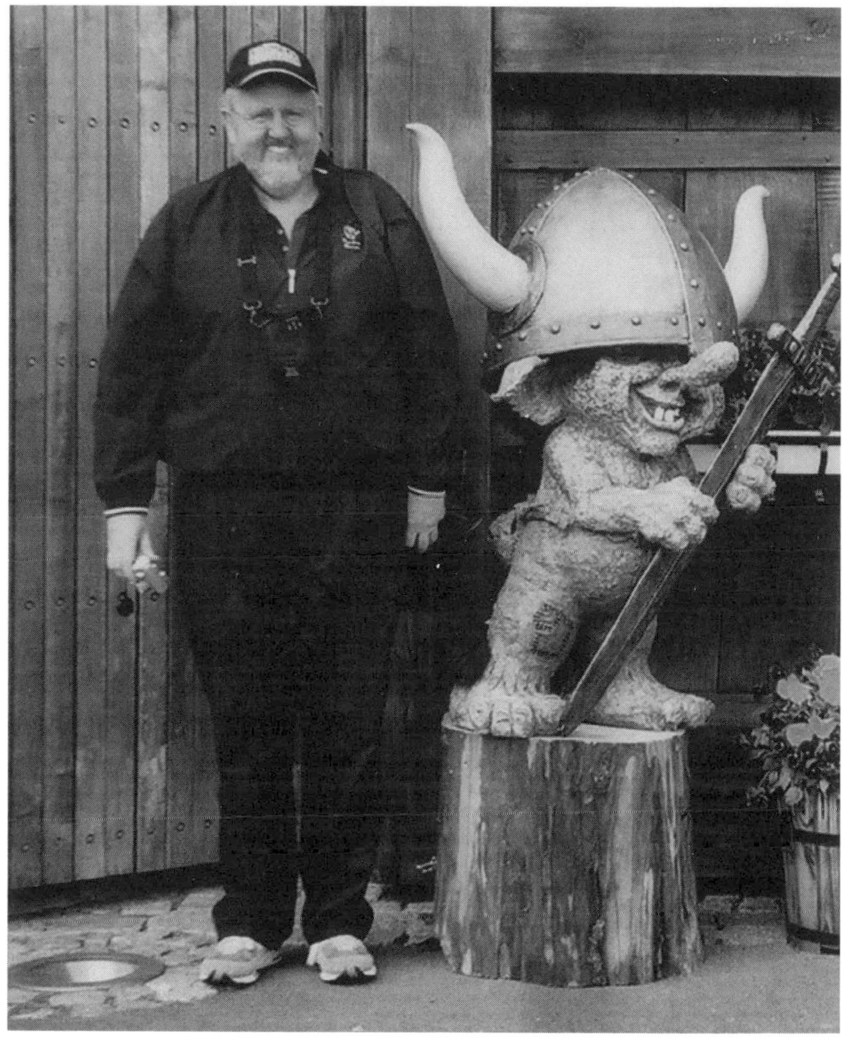

I was on a trip to Norway in 2003, before my scare in New Orleans, when this snapshot was taken. You can see how severely overweight I was.

of the Kirklin Clinic where I worked—a large multi-specialty clinic based at the University of Alabama at Birmingham (UAB). I was quite familiar with those scales, for I had sent my own obese endocrinology patients over to the Geriatric Department to be weighed when they were too heavy for the scales in our office.

I decided to weigh on a Sunday morning, when no one was around. During times when I was on the road for meetings and speaking engagements, it was kind of a standard habit with me that I would go into my office at the Kirklin Clinic on Sundays to catch up on paperwork.

On this particular Sunday morning, it had been several days since I had returned home to Birmingham, Alabama, from my travels to New Orleans and to fulfill my speaking engagements in South Carolina and Pennsylvania. Actually, I already had been back in my office seeing patients for a few days. But I was not about to weigh on a regular-schedule weekday, when the clinic was filled with my physician colleagues, the staff, and patients and their family members and friends. I mean, why would I want anyone around for "My Big Weigh-In"? I didn't want anyone to see!

When I came in that Sunday, things were quiet in the clinic. I had no trouble finding the privacy I wanted for "My Big Weigh-In" on the super-scales at the clinic's Geriatric Department. Since I had planned ahead for this, I had not eaten any breakfast. It had been 12 hours or more since my last meal.

I stepped up on these scales I knew were trustworthy. I looked at what the scales told me. Surprise, surprise!!! It was the second time in two weeks I was stunned in a negative way about a "number" that depicted something associated with my own body. The first surprise of course had been that blood pressure reading in New Orleans. And now here was the second surprise—my weight. Not what I "guessed" my weight would be, but what my weight actually was.

The scales told the sad, ugly truth: 313 pounds! And that was after strict dieting for almost two weeks.

I'll never know for sure what I weighed when I was in New Orleans. It had to be at least 320 pounds. And it easily could have been as much as 325 pounds.

As I stood there looking at 313 pounds showing on those scales in the Kirklin Clinic, I thought, "Well, David, now's your chance. You're an obese man. You're not a well man. All this gives you major motivation. You have reason to get this weight off. So get with it!"

How Much Should I Weigh?

Since I had counseled many of my patients about their own weight, I didn't have to go to any books or the Internet to figure out how much I should weigh.

For my height and body build, I needed to weigh somewhere around 210 pounds. Wow! That was only 103 pounds *less* than the 313 pounds I weighed on that Sunday morning in 2003.

How did I arrive at that target ideal weight of 210?

Well, if an adult male wants to figure his ideal weight, this is the formula he uses: Start with a baseline of five feet in height and a weight of 106 pounds. Then, for every inch, add six pounds. That means a man who is 5 feet, 10 inches tall should weigh roughly 166 pounds.

For a woman to calculate her "ideal weight," she starts with 100 pounds and five feet in height, and she adds five pounds for each inch. This means that a woman of 5 feet, 4 inches would have an "ideal weight" of 120.

Now, this "ideal" can vary as much as 10 percent up or down—depending on how large or small a body frame you have, and frankly, depending on how you look and feel at a given weight.

Since I am a male standing 6 feet, 5 inches in height, that's 17 inches beyond five feet—or 102 pounds. Add the 102 to the base of 106, and you get 208 pounds, if you're going exactly by the "ideal."

I also had to take into account the size body frame I have—which is rather average size. To compute the size of your body frame, measure your wrist—by circling your wrist with your thumb and middle finger. If the thumb and middle finger meet easily around your wrist, you have an average size body frame. If they overlap, you have a small frame. And, if they won't meet, you have a large frame. (In calculating your weight, add an extra 10 percent in pounds if you have a large frame and subtract 10 percent in pounds if you have a small frame.)

In 2003, I set my sights on a target weight for myself that was in the neighborhood of 208 to 210 pounds.

My "Calorie Allowance" for Losing Weight

Since I also had counseled many patients on the *mechanics* of how to lose weight, I knew that the simple ideal answer was to take a two-pronged approach:

◊ Limit the number of calories I took in.

◊ Burn up some of the calories I took in through (1) normal daily activity and also through (2) any exercise regimen that I added.

I knew that my goal was to lose two to two and a half pounds a week. While I realized that was a pretty ambitious goal, I also knew that I was *serious* about this weight-losing project.

To lose two and a half pounds in a week, I needed to have a net intake of no more than roughly 1,600 to 1,800 calories a day.

By "net intake of calories," I mean the total number of daily calories I was left with after (1) adding up all the calories I took in through eating, and (2) subtracting the number of calories I burned up with normal daily activity and exercise.

So how did I arrive at the 1,600-to-1,800 calories a day limit in order for me to lose two and a half pounds in a week?

This is how I figured my "calorie allowance": (You can figure yours the same way.)

◊ You start computing based on your *ideal weight* (not what you weigh when you start your weight-losing program, but instead your ideal weight). To get a baseline for your "calorie allowance," start with your *ideal weight* and multiply by 10. So, back in 2003, since I figured out my ideal weight as 210, I multiplied the 210 pounds by 10 and knew that I started out with a baseline daily calorie allowance of 2,100 calories.

◊ Then you can *add* to your "daily calorie allowance" the number of calories that would be burned up in normal daily activity by the average person of your height and body frame size. As a general rule, you can figure your normal daily activity calories by computing 30 percent of your baseline calorie allowance. In my case, I allowed myself 30 percent of my total daily calorie allowance of 2,100—meaning that I added 630 calories for my daily normal activity. That meant that by adding the 630 calories to my baseline calorie allowance of 2,100, I was now up to a calorie allowance of 2,730 calories a day.

◊ Next you can *add* even more calories to your "daily calorie allowance" by awarding yourself the calories that you will burn in a daily regimen of exercise. The general rule is that for one hour a day of good, healthy exercise—such as an hour of brisk walking—you can give yourself another 500 calories. When I embarked on my weight-loss program in 2003, I made sure I did an hour of daily exercise. So I added 500 calories to my daily calorie allowance. With my baseline of 2,100 calories, plus my normal daily activity allowance of 630 calories, plus my newly added daily exercise regimen of 500 calories, I now was up to a daily calorie allowance of 3,230 calories. When you multiply my daily calorie allowance of 3,230 calories by the seven days in a week, that totals up to my weekly calorie allowance of 22,610.

◊ But, I was wanting to LOSE weight! So now I had to do the tough calculations: I had to take into account how much of that fat I wanted to lose, and I had to start *subtracting* calories. *For every one pound of fat you want to lose in a week, you must subtract 3,600 calories.* A pound of fat is the same in every individual, no matter the person's height, no matter how small or large the body frame, regardless of whether it's a male or female. If I was going to lose two and a half pounds a week, I needed to subtract 3,600 calories for the first pound of fat, and then subtract another 3,600 calories for the second pound of fat, and then subtract another 1,800 calories for a half pound of fat—adding up to a whopping 9,000 calories. To lose an average of two and a half pounds of fat a week, I had to subtract 9,000 calories a week from my weekly calorie allowance of 22,610!

◊ So, by subtracting 9,000 calories from my 22,610 calories, I was left with a weekly calorie allowance of 13,610 calories. That would be 1,944 calories a day.

◊ However, I knew that for me I had to subtract even more calories. The reason had to do with age. The sad truth is that as we get a little older, it's more difficult to lose weight than when we were younger. It's just a fact of life that the body's metabolism slows down with age. This slowdown in body metabolism typically starts at around age 45 in men and around age 35 in women. So, as a 59-year-old man who wanted to lose as much as two and a half pounds in a week, I couldn't expect to do that by eating 1,944 calories a day! That would be more typical of what a guy in his 30s could expect to eat in order to lose that much weight per week. At my age, to meet my goal of losing around two and a half pounds a week, I knew I must drop my daily calorie allowance down to somewhere between 1,600 and 1,800 calories. (I knew if I changed my mind and decided to lose as little as 1 pound a week, I could bump my daily calorie intake up to around 2,500 calories a day. I didn't change my mind about my goal. So I kept the daily calorie intake at around 1,600 to 1,800 a day.)

Giving Some Thought to My New Diet

If you need to lose a substantial amount of weight and keep it off—which certainly was the case with me—then it's important to select a healthy diet plan with which you feel comfortable.

The truth of the matter is that *selecting a diet is in a sense like selecting a spouse.* You *hope* it's a selection for life and *not* just for three or four weeks, or three or four months, or three or four years. (In reality we know that in the U.S. more than 50 percent of marriages end in divorce.) Ideally your diet should be a selection that you can live with for the long-term—actually, for the rest of your life.

As I've told my patients on many occasions, *dieting—like growing older—is not for wimps.* If you're going to be successful in keeping your weight under control, you have to stick to some type of diet plan for a lifetime.

Now, once you are down to your ideal weight, you don't have to be as strict with your diet as you were when you were losing the weight. But if you don't maintain some consistent, ongoing dietary discipline, if you don't stick to your diet plan in a realistically modified way even after you have lost weight, then that weight will creep right back on again.

Since I had lost weight several times in the past and had regained the weight every time, I knew from personal experience that I really needed a diet that I *liked,* a diet that I actually found appealing. So I really gave some thought to a diet that I thought would work for me—a diet I could come to enjoy and view as a friend and a partner.

Selecting One Meal a Day

The diet component of my diet/exercise regimen that I settled on was that I would eat only one meal a day. I decided that each day I would eat one balanced meal with reasonable portions of food.

While this one-meal-a-day might sound a bit drastic to some folks, it's a diet that I thought out carefully and settled on for five key reasons. The reasons that applied when I started the diet in 2003 still apply today. With very slight modifications, I'm still using the one-meal-a-day diet in order to maintain my ideal weight. Not only is it working for me; I also enjoy it!

MY FIVE REASONS for deciding on the one-meal-a-day approach:

1. I found the one-meal-a-day to be *historically appealing.* I was drawn to it by its historical context with our ancestors. I still am.

2. I felt the one-meal-a-day plan would be *effective* in losing weight and keeping it off. For me it indeed has been effective in losing weight and keeping it off.

3. I felt the one-meal-a-day plan would be *healthy.* I believe it has been extremely healthy for me. My "numbers" are great (blood pressure, cholesterol, blood sugar levels, etc.) And I feel great!

4. I felt the one-meal-a-day plan would be *time-pacing.* It has been, and it is, in very positive ways.

5. I felt the one-meal-a-day plan would be *enjoyable.* It was, and it still is.

The Historical Appeal of One Meal a Day

I found the one-meal-a-day concept to be appealing because of a link this concept has to the history of our ancestors and their lifestyles relevant to eating.

You know, this whole habit that we have of eating three meals a day has somewhat evolved over the centuries. In the lives of primitive man, families didn't spend all day eating. They basically ate one meal a day.

When our ancestors got up early in the morning, they did not eat. Instead, they went out on their daily missions of finding something to eat, by gathering and hunting. The women went out collecting nuts and berries. The men went out hunting. In the evening, the family members came together and "shared their spoils" so to speak. They had one main meal a day—one feast.

In modern-day times, our own bodies and the needs of our bodies are the same as they were with primitive man. Our bodies are really not adapted to eating multiple meals per day. Our genetics are not really programmed to accept all this food.

Since our bodies and the needs of our bodies have not changed, what is it that has changed? The answer is simple: Our lifestyles have changed; the food-related choices that we make in our lifestyles have changed. Generations after generations in our society have gradually changed lifestyles over the centuries to accommodate more and more food. We've decided that we need to eat more often, that we need to eat the wrong things, and that we need to eat larger amounts of those wrong things.

The Effectiveness of One Meal a Day

I looked at the one-meal-a-day regimen as a choice for me because I knew it would be effective in controlling my intake of calories.

If you're trying to lose a substantial amount of weight and keep it off, I think that goal can be very difficult, and often impossible, to attain while eating three meals a day. Too, if you somehow manage to lose a lot of weight while eating three meals a day, quite often those "meals" are so skimpy that you never, ever leave the table satisfied.

I just felt plain and simply that it seemed an effective idea to me to "put all my eggs in one basket" as the old saying goes. In putting all my eggs in one basket, I have been able to eat one meal a day consisting of food I really enjoy.

The Health Benefits of One Meal a Day

From time to time over the years, I had patients come to me who ate only one meal a day. I particularly remember some patients of Italian descent who preferred the one-meal-a-day approach. Two impressions struck me about these patients: Number one, they consistently kept their weight down. And, number two, overall they were very healthy people.

It's not at all uncommon for senior citizens to eat mainly one meal a day. In fact, sometimes a new resident in a senior-living facility will have trouble adjusting to the facility's routine of three meals a day.

If someone comes to me and says, "I think one meal a day sounds unhealthy," I will respond that "I am convinced one meal a day is quite the opposite; I believe one meal a day is an extremely healthy way to eat." For example, it has recently been shown that the greater the volume of fat in the liver, the lower the production of HDL (good cholesterol). The amount of fat in the liver *decreases* with fasting. Therefore, eating once daily may result not only in increased HDL but also in a greater protection against cardiovascular events (heart attack, stroke, etc.).

I'm not saying that every individual out there has a health situation that lends itself to eating one meal a day. There's not a diet plan on the planet that is universal enough to match everyone's health needs and personal preferences. But, as one who has studied and treated metabolic conditions for decades, I will tell you that there are many, many individuals out there who can lead much healthier lives by eating just one meal a day.

Before anyone starts a diet and exercise program, the person needs to check with his or her personal physician. That's just a given. If you are embarking on a major weight-loss program, it's *essential* that you seek out expert medical advice about how your own health status matches with whatever weight-loss program you are considering. When you discuss this with your physician, he or she might say that my one-meal-a-day plan would work well for you. Or your physician might say that you have health issues that do not match the one-meal-a day plan.

Now, having strongly flagged your obtaining an expert medical opinion about yourself as a *must*, I will share with you, in general terms, some of my strong views as a physician about one-meal-a-day. These are views that you can discuss with your own physician in relation to you and one meal a day: I can tell you that there are many individuals with diabetes who can use the one-meal-a-day approach. I can tell you that I believe many heart attacks can be prevented if more people would eat one sensible meal a day instead of gorging themselves with three meals, many of them heavy. The time after a meal—particularly a heavy meal—is a very risky time for heart attacks, because the elevation of glucose and fats in the blood can actually lead to a heart attack. This is especially true following a heavy, fatty breakfast! One group of individuals who are at particular risk for suffering a heart attack following a heavy meal are men in general—especially of course those men who also have other risk factors. Another group of individuals who are at high risk for suffering a heart attack after a heavy meal are both men and women who have diabetes. So it stands to reason that if you consume fewer meals, and if you design those meals with wise food selections and reasonable portions, you can cut back on the risk of heart attacks.

Note: Chapter 9 in this book contains more about how the one-meal-a-day approach can apply to you and your loved ones.

The Time-Pacing Nature of One Meal a Day

Eating one meal a day is a great "time pacer" in two respects: (1) paving the way for more leisurely eating during one meal, while at the same time (2) cutting down on overall time spent eating. This is how it works:

On the one hand, eating one meal a day encourages you to avoid "rushing your eating" and instead to devote more quality time to the one meal a day than you ordinarily would tend to do. (Rushing food tends to increase your food intake.)

On the other hand, even when you devote a bit more time to that one meal, you'll still tend to spend less time overall related to eating. By sticking to one meal a day, you will tend to net some hours in your days.

◊ **Not rushing that one meal.** There is no doubt in my mind than when you eat that one meal a day you are likely to eat it slowly and thoughtfully. By eating slowly and thoughtfully, you are less likely to just sit there and cram food in your mouth without really thinking about how much you're eating and what you're eating. Here's the theory, and I know it worked for me: That one meal has become special to me. I plan what I'm going to eat. I take time to enjoy what I eat. I don't just shovel in food without thinking. Even if I'm having conversations with dinner companions, I make sure that I eat more slowly than I did in the past, that I eat less than in the past, and that I enjoy my food more than in the past. The benefits I derive? For one thing, when I don't rush food, I tend to take in fewer calories. For another thing, eating slower is better for my digestive system, better for my metabolism. Quick equals too much!

Note: Chapter 9 contains more about how you can reduce your calorie intake by not rushing food and also by not being distracted by work or other stimuli when you're eating.

◊ **Saving time overall:** Many of us complain that we never have enough time to do the things we need to do and want to do. At work we often can't cram in all the tasks in front of us. In our personal lives, for lack-of-time reasons we often delay for months visiting with friends and family members that we really want to see. And what about having a little time for ourselves—to read a good book, to work in the garden, to catch that movie that our friends say is so great?

I have found it a true gift to have the extra time I've been given by eating only one meal a day. If we think about the enormous amounts of time that go into the three-meals-a-day habit, we can be amazed at how many hours we spend procuring, preparing, and eating all that food—and often also in cleaning up after ourselves after we eat. I can personally attest that this "bonus" time that has come my way can be put to use in other constructive ways. (Oh, and by the way, you not only can save time with one meal a day; you can save some money along the way as well.)

The Enjoyment of One Meal a Day

I'll have to admit that the pure "enjoyment" angle was a big draw in my decision to eat only one meal a day.

I love good food. And even though I was going on a serious diet, I didn't want to give up the enjoyment of good food. For me, that meant that I did not want to go through the day looking at three meals of meager portions of something I didn't want, and always having to think about what I was doing without. (And maybe then still not losing weight!)

Instead, I wanted my diet to be a positive one. I wanted to be able to look forward to one time a day when I could have reasonable portions of good, healthy food. That's what I got. And it has worked.

I'll tell you one thing: Since I began my one-meal-a-day lifestyle, I no longer have taken eating for granted. During that one meal a day, I have learned to eat more slowly, to think about what I'm eating, to really taste the food and appreciate it.

Through eating one meal a day, I have found more enjoyment than I ever did in eating three meals a day in years gone by. No, let's be honest here: I have found more enjoyment in eating one meal a day than I did during my past habit of eating three meals a day PLUS, PLUS, PLUS!!

One Meal a Day Draws Some Questions

From the time I "let the cat out of the bag" and described my "One-Plus-One Plan" to a few family members and friends, I began hearing some of the same questions about the one-meal-a-day component of my plan.

These are some of the most frequently-asked questions—followed by some answers:

◊ What were you eating prior to starting your one meal a day?

◊ What do you typically eat now at your one meal a day?

◊ Do you totally eliminate carbohydrates from your diet?

◊ What time of day do you eat your one meal a day?

◊ Who are your eating companions now that you eat only one meal a day?

What I Was Eating "Before"

After a person loses a great deal or weight, keeps it off, and feels good about this success, it can be a bit mind-boggling for that person to go back and recall what he or she was eating "before"—as in before the weight loss.

I have spoken over the years to patients who had that experience. Then, in 2003 and 2004 I became one of those people.

As painful as it is—and a bit embarrassing as well—let's review some typical aspects of my eating habits prior to June 2003.

Breakfast: I actually had a fairly light breakfast—like a couple of slices of toast, a glass of orange juice, and a cup of coffee. (As an aside about this whole matter of eating breakfast: For some reason, many obese people tend to start out the day eating little or no breakfast, but then indulge themselves on large amounts of food as the day goes along.)

After breakfast, things started going downhill for me. Downhill, that is, in terms of my using common sense with my eating. *Uphill* in terms of how much I ate.

When I was in town on weekdays, I generally consumed my lunch while at work at the Kirklin Clinic. While my lunch menu tended to vary a bit, it usually was high in calories and fat. Often I attended a lunch meeting. There always was plenty of food at those meetings, and I got my share of it! There also were days when representatives of pharmaceutical firms would bring in lunch for us to eat while we discussed new medications. Those meals tended to be quite ample and also very high in calories. Then there were the days when I would venture to a deli conveniently located near my office. At the deli I typically purchased one of those sandwiches that on the surface looked pretty healthy, except for all that mayonnaise and heavy bread—a lot of calories. And, oh yes, I usually would follow the sandwich with some ice cream, yogurt, or something even worse. Suffice it to say I was not into discreet, light lunches.

Then came what for me was the Biggest Meal of the Day—the evening meal. Virtually every night I would badly overeat. First I would have a generous serving of everything we were having in the main course—meat, rice, vegetables, whatever. Then generally I would go back and have a second serving of all that. Most evenings I ate an awful lot of bread. (Ever since my early childhood, I had eaten an awful lot of bread.) If cheese was around, I would eat a lot of cheese. I've always liked cheese. Now, eating cheese is not so bad if you don't overdo it; cheese is quite filling and does tend to suppress the appetite. But obviously it was not suppressing my appetite, and I would eat a lot of cheese on top of everything else. Then there were the desserts. We had desserts most every evening—heavy, sweet desserts, such as a pie or a cake. I would always have dessert. And more often than not, I would have two helpings of dessert. I can recall on many an evening after dinner that I would sit down and feel so stuffed. I sometimes would tell myself something to the effect of: "You are just loaded with food! You've really overeaten. This is not good." Then the next night I would do it all over again.

What I Eat Now

Now that I'm eating only one meal a day, I consume mainly meats, vegetables, and low-sugar fruits, some carbohydrate but not a whole lot, and no traditional sweet desserts.

In my one daily meal, I eat a balanced meal that is a modified version of the evening meal I ate prior to starting my diet. My one meal typically consists of reasonable portions of a meat, a couple of vegetables, perhaps a salad with low-calorie dressing, and sometimes a bit of fruit or cheese in the place of a dessert.

These are some adjustments I have made in what once was my evening meal.

◊ **Portions:** I eat reasonable portions of food, and I don't go back for "seconds."

◊ **Bread:** If I allow myself any bread, it's a very small amount of bread. When I was still in the process of losing weight, I cut out most of the bread. Now that I'm in a program to maintain my ideal weight rather than lose more weight, I allow myself a bit more bread than when I was really dieting, but still not much. I know that bread is my biggest food downfall. I have to be very careful there.

◊ **Desserts:** I no longer eat any conventional sweet desserts, and I don't plan to start back eating them. That means no pies, no cakes, no ice cream, etc. I've found that I do well with substituting a piece of low-sugar fruit or some cheese. (*Note*: In Chapter 9, I elaborate on these dessert substitutes.)

◊ **Beverages:** Where beverages are concerned, I steer away from sweet beverages. Since I've lost down to my ideal weight, I occasionally allow myself a glass of wine with dinner. However, I'm careful that I don't drink that glass of wine before dinner on an empty stomach, for then I would be setting the stage for the wine to quickly go to my head and lower my blood sugar, thus stimulating my appetite.

Note: In Chapter 9, I'll have more advice to offer about healthy eating habits for dieters—including some discussion about my own favorite foods and also about those same old 20 foods that most people eat!

A Word about Carbohydrates and Me

Even though I limit carbohydrates in my diet, I do consume a small amount of carbohydrates. I am strongly opposed to these diets that call for absolutely no carbohydrates.

Our bodies are not geared to be totally deprived of carbohydrates. That's unnatural, and the body can rebel. Too, if you go on one of these no-carbohydrate diets, it's not likely you'll be able to sustain it on the long-term and the weight will just come back.

I believe that it's beneficial to weight-loss and beneficial to healthy well-being to consume low amounts, controlled amounts, of carbohydrates. At the same time, I think the total elimination of carbohydrates can have side effects that range from unpleasant to unhealthy to downright dangerous.

As a physician, I have seen patients experience some of the following side effects after going on diets that totally eliminate carbohydrates from the diet:

◊ **A rise in cholesterol levels—particularly a rise in the LDL cholesterol, which we have come to call the "bad cholesterol."** There's just no doubt that these no-carbohydrate diets place many dieters at risk for cholesterol hikes. The reason is that when you shift from eating carbohydrates to eating a large amount of protein, along with that protein you are likely to take in a lot of fat (such as through fatty meats that are high in protein). And the increased fat intake can translate into higher levels of the bad cholesterol. Individuals at particularly high risk for this complication are those we call "high absorbers of fat." I'm referring to the fact that there are certain people who will *dramatically* increase their cholesterol while on a high-fat diet because they tend to absorb much more fat than is normal or average. Unfortunately we can't predict which individual will or won't be a high absorber of fat.

◊ **Disruption in normal metabolism.** Eating too little carbohydrate can set the stage for a metabolic state called "ketosis." In ketosis, there is an abnormal breakdown of fat in the body, and a rise in organic compounds called "ketones." This can result in a very unhealthy metabolic state for your body. For example, this situation can make your body far too acid, creating a state we simply call "acidosis." If your body experiences this high-acid condition over a long period, if you have chronic acidosis, this condition can put you at risk for thinning of the bones, or osteoporosis.

◊ **Hair loss.** Some of my physician colleagues and I have encountered individuals whose hair started falling out after they totally deprived the body of carbohydrates. I know one man who had thick, longish hair when he started his no-carb diet and who had very thin hair when he finished it. Although he lost 55 pounds on a no-carbohydrate diet, he shed his hair along with shedding the pounds! It is my belief that his hair loss was directly related to "ketosis," which in turn was a direct result of the man having eliminated carbohydrates from his diet.

◊ **A very unpleasant fruity-smelling breath.** If you're around someone who has a very fruity-smelling breath and the person tells you he or she is on a no-carbohydrate diet, you can be pretty sure the fruity breath and the diet are connected. This breath smell can be quite unpleasant, kind of a nasty fruity smell. It has an odor somewhat like the breath of someone who has been consuming alcohol heavily.

◊ **A sluggish feeling.** People on no-carbohydrate diets often simply do not feel well. The no-carb dieter is not providing his or her body with the balance of nutrients it needs to maintain energy, stamina, and an overall feeling of well-being.

◊ **Severe constipation.** The body's mechanics for eliminating wastes are interrupted with a no-carb diet. Normal bowel movements can become less frequent and more difficult when they do occur.

◊ **Heart arrhythmias.** Problems with irregular heartbeat are among the more dangerous side effects that have been seen in some patients on no-carbohydrate diets.

I've lost a lot of weight, and I'm keeping the weight off. But all along the way—when I was losing weight, and now that I'm maintaining the weight—I have been *very* focused on including a controlled amount of carbohydrates in my diet.

The Time of Day I Eat My One Meal a Day

I generally eat my one meal a day in the early evening. I selected that time because it works with my lifestyle. When I'm on the road with speaking engagements and meetings, I usually can work it into the schedule to have time to really enjoy an early evening meal. When I'm home, it's important to me to eat my one meal whenever possible with my wife, Jocelyn. And early evening works for her.

If someone were to ask me the absolutely ideal time to eat only one meal a day—from the standpoint of losing weight, and likely also from a health viewpoint—my answer would be "without question, in the morning—the breakfast meal." The reason is that your metabolism is at its peak first thing in the morning, and your body is going to use up calories more efficiently with a morning meal.

Actually, if you select one meal a day and stick with it, you're going to lose weight no matter what time of day you eat. Some people will be happier eating in the middle of the day. I think most, however, would select the evening—because our culture is so geared to eating in the evening.

Now, if I could eat at absolutely the hour of the day that I prefer, I would pick four o'clock in the afternoon. That's early enough in the day to be a daytime meal, and it's late enough in the day to be an evening meal. It's early enough in the day so that you don't get too hungry during the day before you eat, and thus you're not tempted to overeat. It's late enough in the day so that you're not likely to get hungry before you go to bed. However, with my schedule it's usually between 5 and 6 P.M. when I eat, sometimes even later.

My Eating Companions

When someone asks me about my eating companions, my answer is this: *"The question is not so much who I eat with as my rule against being around other people who are eating when I'm not eating!"*

You see, my self-discipline about food consumption does have its limits. I've found that in order to maintain my diet, I simply do not generally place myself in the presence of people who are eating when I'm *not* eating."

I don't say any of this in jest. I'm serious about this. One of the keys to the success of my diet plan is that I don't sit around and watch other people eat when I'm not eating. I steer away from that whenever possible—and will always do so. I must do that, because if I'm around other people who are eating I am very likely going to want to eat, too. That's the way I think. I'm not in a boat by myself with this thinking. That's the way obese people in general tend to think about food. Even though I am now thin in size, I still have the attitude about food that obese people tend to have. I was obese so long (most all my life) that I likely will always think like an obese person in relation to food and eating. There still is a fat person deep inside me. Thus I will always try to steer clear of people who are eating when I am not eating.

Let me explain this: If you're thin, you are likely to want to eat when you get physical signs that you are hungry—like maybe when you are feeling a bit weak or shaky, or your stomach is contracting, maybe "growling," maybe even cramping a bit. Not so if you're obese! If you're an obese person, the stimuli that tell you that you want to eat will be different. As an obese person, you'll want to eat at the very sight or thought of food—even if you've just eaten and your stomach is full. You'll want to eat if you see someone else eating. You'll want to eat if you smell food. You'll want to eat if you see food advertised on television. You'll want to eat if the clock tells you it's time for you to eat—even if you've been eating off and on all day.

Actually, this whole eating mindset of obese people is why "fat farms" tend to work so well—or at least why fat farms work as long as the obese person is confined to the fat farm. At fat farms, the obese person is removed from food to a great degree. So the obese person loses weight. Then, after the obese person is mainstreamed back into society and around food once again, he or she is very likely to gain back the weight—unless the person recognizes these tendencies and makes adjustments.

Now, since I was aware of the stimuli that motivated obese people when I started my weight-loss program back in 2003, I took steps accordingly.

Take my situation at home, for example. My wife, Jocelyn, does not stick to one meal per day. Although she and I eat the evening meal together when I'm home, Jocelyn usually eats apart from me at lunch-time.

For whatever reason, watching Jocelyn eat breakfast doesn't bother me. Maybe that's because I never ate much breakfast anyhow. At any rate, while Jocelyn is eating breakfast, I'm having a cup of coffee. And I'm fine with that. However, watching Jocelyn eat lunch can bother me and cause me to want to eat, too. It is typical for Jocelyn to have a salad or sandwich for lunch. More often than not, I'll go to another room while she's eating her lunch salad or sandwich. I simply do not want to see Jocelyn's lunch food when I'm not eating. I'm an obese person in the way I react, and I don't want to see her lunch food because it makes me hungry. On the other hand, if I don't see Jocelyn or someone else eating lunch, I'm not hungry in the middle of the day. I'm fine until I sit down for my one meal a day in the evening.

When it comes time for my one meal a day in the evening, I welcome someone to join me and share the meal experience with me. When I'm eating my one meal a day, I usually have companions at the meal—Jocelyn, other family members and friends, or, when I'm on the road, professional colleagues with whom I'm meeting or to whom I'm making clinical presentations.

The Exercise Component of the One-Plus-One Plan

When it came to the exercise component of my One-Plus-One Weight-Loss Plan, I didn't have to make as many drastic changes in my lifestyle as I did with the dieting component.

Needless to say, in the several years preceding the year 2003, I had not been on any kind of calorie-limiting diet. However, I had been getting at least *some* physical exercise.

I was on and off with the exercising. Sometimes I would be real good about it, and other times I would not be. In short, the exercise was spotty, inconsistent, not enough. But at least it was something.

Prior to launching my weight-loss program, the inconsistent exercise that I did consisted mainly of my on-again/off-again walking program.

Too, there had been times in my home when I had used first one treadmill and then another for exercise. However, the treadmills I had bought for the house were far too cheap and couldn't take the abuse I gave them. One after another, the treadmills broke down and moved on out of my life.

When I launched my weight-loss program, I took stock of where I was with exercise. I set about the task of expanding the exercise—with the goal of coming up with an hour a day of consistent, healthy exercise.

It took a while for me to settle on just the right exercise regimen for me. It actually took a while for me to become consistent with one hour a day of exercise.

On this exercise journey, I went through three stages:

◊ The walking stage.

◊ The treadmill stage, with some walking.

◊ The treadmill and weights stage, with some walking.

The Walking Stage

For years I have believed that the best exercise you can get is brisk walking. I still believe that. If you just walk briskly, you're not likely to damage your back, your knees, your ankles, or your feet.

Just don't carry weights when you walk. I am totally against that. Walking while carrying hand weights or while wearing weights on your legs or other parts of your body can be very destructive to your joints.

At the same time I started eating one meal a day to cut back on calories, I also made a concerted effort to expand the amount of time I walked and to do it every day.

I walked some in the malls. I like walking in the malls. There you have air-conditioning. That's important in the Deep South where I live, with the high heat and high humidity in the summer months (and some other months as well). Also in the malls you can be nice and dry. The Deep South tends to have its share of rainy days as well as its share of hot, humid days.

Weather permitting, some days I walked outdoors. When the weather is nice, one thing about walking in the Birmingham area is that the scenery can be very pleasant. I would walk on very scenic trails a few miles from my home, or I would walk in my neighborhood.

However, when I walked in my neighborhood I often had some unwelcome "companions." I frequently encountered dogs that would come after me and go straight for my ankles. This occurred despite the fact there allegedly is a leash law in effect in our area. (Actually, the bothersome dogs would come after both me and my own dog, who was just walking along with me while minding her own business and making absolutely no move to bother any fellow canines.)

With the demanding patient-care schedule I had in 2003, the most practical time for me to try to walk on weekdays was in the late afternoon or early evening. However, with work-schedule reality what it was, I found that sometimes I arrived home too late to do the walking. I often would return home from work long after the sun went down, when it was so dark outside that I felt I should not be outdoors walking. And sometimes by the time I could go to the malls at night, the malls were closed up and locked for the night.

By late 2003, after I had been on my weight-loss program for a full six months, it seemed to me that the obstacles to my walking program were mounting. With the weather issue, and the dog issue, and my own hours not matching with shopping mall hours, I was in the market for a new program of exercise.

"Midnight Madness" and a New Treadmill

Although women have more of a reputation for shopping sprees than do men, I had my own exercise-related shopping spree of sorts in December 2003.

One night when Jocelyn and I were returning from a Christmas party, we were driving by a store that had a sign advertising a "Midnight Madness Sale." The store had exercise equipment on sale. On impulse, I went into the store, looked around at the exercise equipment, and proceeded to spot a good bargain in a really high-quality treadmill. However, even at a good bargain it was more money than I would think of spending on a piece of exercise equipment. I believe I still was in a mindset of my longstanding habits of on-again, off-again exercise. I think I was hearing a voice inside me asking, "Now, are you *really* going to use this expensive thing enough to justify this investment??? Or will you just use the treadmill as a handy place where you can hang your clothes?"

By the next morning, when it came time for me to return to the store to pick up my purchase, I had changed my mind. I told Jocelyn, "I don't think I'm going through with this purchase. I don't really need that treadmill. I'm not going to get it."

I quickly found that one member of the Bell family had not had a change of heart. Jocelyn said, "Yes, you're going to get it."

This was just another in a series of positive reactions from Jocelyn that helped drive forward my weight-loss program.

As you will recall, it was Jocelyn's concern about my overweight condition and her fears about my health status that led me to get my blood pressure checked in New Orleans and find out I had high blood pressure.

Then, when I embarked on my program of eating only one meal a day, Jocelyn supported that. She was very willing to help me even though it changed her life as well. She supported my new eating pattern even though it slightly changed the time of day she served our evening meal (by scheduling that meal a bit earlier in the evening). She supported my new eating pattern even though it somewhat changed the menu she planned for our evening meal (mainly eliminating those tasty desserts). And she supported my one-meal-a-day plan even though my new eating routine often meant that Jocelyn ate her lunch alone in one room while I stayed in another room—to accommodate my need to avoid watching others eat when I was not eating.

So, when it came to my setting up a program to exercise an hour a day, Jocelyn was very supportive there as well. She wanted me to have a convenient way to exercise. And she believed buying the new treadmill was a good idea.

So the new treadmill was purchased and brought home as a welcomed addition to the Bell household.

I'll have to say that adding the treadmill solved my exercise issues. From the day I brought that treadmill into our home, it has been my ticket to getting a full hour of exercise every day. While I'm exercising on the treadmill, I often enjoy watching news programs on television or movies or DVDs.

In addition to the treadmill exercising, when the weather is nice there are some days when I still get out and walk—if I can steer clear of the dogs, that is. But rain or shine, no matter what time I get home, the treadmill has become the central core of my exercise program.

Adding the Weights

When you're losing weight—particularly a great deal of weight—I think you need to monitor yourself and you may find that it helps to "tweak" parts of your weight-loss program as you see the need.

In the latter part of 2003 and on into 2004, the pounds began to drop off my once-very-bulky body. I was pleased. However, in "monitoring" myself, I realized that my upper body began looking a little thin and puny. Jocelyn commented on this, as did a few of my friends.

So I decided it was time to add to my daily routine some weight-lifting exercises to strengthen and build muscle in my upper body.

Before starting any kind of exercises with weights, I consulted someone I knew who already had experience in this area—the middle of our three sons, Michael. I told him, "Michael, I need to gain some upper body bulk. So tell me what to do." Michael seemed delighted. For he had to look no further for a Christmas-gift idea for his father. He said, "I'll get you a Christmas present!" And he did.

Thus, just as the treadmill came into my life in the month of December (2003), the weights also were added in the month of December (2004). Michael got me a workbench, and two weights each of 5 pounds, 10 pounds and 20 pounds. Michael also showed me how to use the weights.

The exercises I do with the weights are all related to my upper-body and abdominal areas. I do exercises for the biceps and triceps (upper arm), deltoids (shoulder area), and pectorals (chest). While I always do either the treadmill or the walking every day, I don't do weights every day. I do the weights maybe three or four days a week, for about 15 minutes a session.

After I added the weights to my exercise program, I soon began seeing positive changes in the upper part of my body. I started to build muscle, and I no longer had that "puny" look.

While some people will say that you'll gain back some weight if you start building muscle with exercise, that was not my experience. Actually, I *lost* a few more pounds after I added the weights to my exercise program and started building muscle. My theory is that while on the one hand you're adding muscle, on the other hand you're burning calories while exercising with those weights.

Making Arrangements to Exercise "On the Road"

As much as I travel to make clinical presentations (and some traveling for pleasure as well), I knew that any daily exercise program would have to include a plan for exercising "on the road."

I knew what I needed in order to make that plan happen. I added something to my criteria for selecting a hotel. Whenever lodging reservations are being made, I check to locate a hotel that has a workout room with a treadmill.

All in all, I've had mixed experience with these hotel workout rooms. Some have very up-to-date treadmills that work beautifully, and they have a pleasant workout room with a comfortable room temperature. In other cases, I've found workout rooms with very worn treadmills that have loose belts, and I've found workout rooms that were far too hot or far too cold.

But I've trudged ahead in using these hotel workout rooms. After all, the only piece of exercise equipment I use in these hotel exercise rooms is the treadmill. For weight-bearing exercises, I prefer the set of weights that Michael gave me.

There are occasions when I'm traveling that I'll mix my treadmill exercise in with a bit of walking. However, I only go walking when I'm already familiar with a walking trail in the city or town I'm visiting, or when someone I trust recommends and describes a good, safe walking trail to me. That's something I'm very careful about, and I would urge all individuals to take care. When you walk, know and be aware of your surroundings. Exercise is a must. It's also a must that you be safe when you exercise.

Chapter 3

WHO CAN USE THIS PLAN?

Since I've lost weight on this plan, and have managed to keep it off, I've had many people come to me and quiz me about who *can* and who *cannot* use the plan and how they can, or cannot, modify it.

This is a sampling of some questions that have come my way—and my answers:

The Main Target Group

Question: When you devised this weight-loss plan, what group of people did you mainly have in mind who should use the plan?

Answer: I devised this weight-loss plan for people who have a significant weight problem—that is, those who are 20 percent or more over their ideal weight. Now, with the overweight problem we have in this nation, there are hundreds of thousands of individuals who would fall into this category.

Frankly, I see no reason for thin people to be on this plan.

Since the obesity problem in this country also includes an ever-increasing number of children, I do feel that many children could benefit from this weight-loss plan, or from some modified version of it. Before parents place their child on this plan, they should consult the child's physician.

I'm big on that advice: Don't embark on this plan, or any other, before you consult a physician who understands you and your own individual health history.

Those "Old Nutrition Rules" We've Always Heard

Question: If this eating-one-meal-a-day plan is really healthy, then what about the adages we've always heard that "You need to eat three balanced meals a day" and "You must have a healthy breakfast to get your day off to a good start"?

Answer: For healthy eating, the important thing is that you daily consume a total intake of foods that gives you the vitamins and minerals you need. It's not important *when* you consume those foods during the day. Also, from a health standpoint, it's not important whether you divide your daily food intake into two meals or three meals or even five or six meals, or *whether you choose to go by this plan and consume all of your daily food intake in one meal.* In choosing what you eat in your daily food intake—and that goes for one meal a day as well—you must consume a balance of lean meat (protein), fruits, vegetables, nuts, minimal carbohydrate, and dairy products for Vitamin D. (And, to lose weight, remember to *limit* your calorie intake. A basic premise of this one-meal-a-day part of my plan is that you will consume fewer calories if you eat only one well-balanced, calorie-controlled meal per day.)

Where did the concept come from that you have to eat three times a day for good-health? I have no idea. And I don't subscribe to that.

Where did the concept come from that you have to eat a good breakfast? I have no idea. There is no medical evidence I've ever seen that people have to eat in the morning in order to be healthy. Many people don't want to eat in the morning; and if they don't want to eat in the morning, they should not feel they have to push themselves to eat in the morning in order to be healthy.

This Plan and Special Health Issues—Such as Diabetes

Question: What about this one-meal-a-day plan for people who have special health issues, such as individuals with diabetes?

Answer: Again—and I can't stress this enough—anyone who wants to go on this weight-loss program (or any other weight-loss program) should first get it cleared through his or her physician. That holds true for *anyone;* it particularly holds true *for those who have known health issues.*

Having said that, I will say from my experience as a longtime internal-medicine specialist, and as a *subspecialist* in metabolism and diabetes care, that many individuals who have special health issues can use this plan and

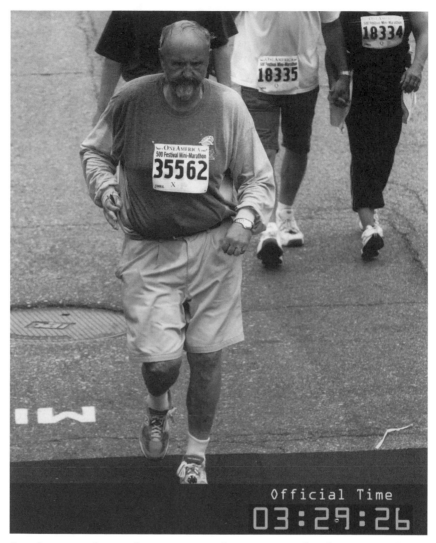

I can't overemphasize the importance of exercise. But I'm also an example that it's never too late to start. In May 2007 in Indianapolis, I finished a half-marathon—a little over 13 miles—in less than three and a half hours.

can benefit from the results.

That includes many individuals with diabetes. Now, there will be some individuals who cannot use this plan—including diabetes patients who have chronic problems with low blood sugar. However, I would recommend this plan to many of my own patients I have treated over the years for diabetes—as long as they do not have chronic low-blood-sugar problems and as long as they are on medicines *that do not tend to cause low-blood sugar*. (Those medicines that do not tend to cause low blood sugar include Metformin®, Avandia®, Actose®, Acarbose®, Miglitol®, Januvia®, and Byetta®.)

Again, check first with your own physician about your own situation.

A Modified Version of the Plan

Question: If a person wants to use this diet, but just can't stick consistently to the one-meal-a-day routine, is there any in-between program that still can be a help?

Answer: My answer is that a little bit of improvement is better than no improvement at all. So, by all means you can modify my plan somewhat and still get some good results.

If you think you absolutely cannot make it on one meal a day, try one of the following:

Just drop one meal. In eating your other two daily meals, keep your choice of foods balanced and healthy and your calorie intake low.

Eat one main healthy meal, and, in addition, treat yourself to a low-calorie snack—or even to *two* low-calorie snacks—at whenever time or times you choose during the day. To make this a bit easier for you—and for better results in weight loss—focus on eating some foods along the way (including your snacks) that make you fill full—so-called "high-satiety," low-calorie foods, such as apples or nuts.

If you have a really significant weight problem, I would still recommend that you gradually "evolve" into eating just one meal a day.

How Important Is This Exercise Thing?

Question: Does a person really need to exercise to make this program work well?

Answer: Yes!! Calorie restriction and exercise go hand in hand. One without the other will not be successful.

Chapter 4

How Good It Is!

As the weeks and months went by in late 2003 and early 2004, I continued to shed pounds. The more pounds I shed, the better I felt—physically and mentally.

By late Spring of 2004—11 months after I started my diet—I was down to my target weight. Actually, I got down to 10 pounds *below* my target weight. I weighed 200 pounds. That was 113 pounds less than when I first weighed in June 2003.

Since I likely had lost between 7 and 12 pounds in the two weeks before I weighed, I calculate the total weight loss at between 120 and 125 pounds. If you figure about 48 weeks from the beginning of my weight-loss program and calculate a weight loss of 120 pounds, I actually had lost at around my goal of 2½ pounds a week.

There was a general consensus—among some family members and friends and myself—that I probably had lost a bit more than I needed to. I had a gaunt look about me. So I set about gradually gaining back 10 pounds. That leveled me off at 210 pounds, where I've been ever since. (I've kept it off, for four years now!!!) It feels good.

I'm not sure words are adequate to describe How Good It Is—in so many ways.

My life is better in terms of the following and more:

- ◊ A more optimistic feeling about my health and well-being.
- ◊ Feeling better, having more energy to live and enjoy life.
- ◊ Sleeping better—a better night's sleep for me *and* for my wife.
- ◊ An improved personal self-image.
- ◊ An improved professional self-image.

◊ And, believe it or not with all this dieting, an *increased* enjoyment of food!

My Health and Well-Being

From that day in June 2003 in New Orleans when I learned that I had dangerously high blood pressure, I've never lost sight of the reason I embarked on this weight-loss program in the first place. I decided to lose 100 pounds-plus for health reasons.

As a result of my diet and exercise program, today I have a much better outlook about my health and well-being. My blood pressure is under control. My other "numbers" are in line, including cholesterol and blood sugar levels. In fact, my good cholesterol (HDL) is higher than my bad cholesterol (LDL).

I believe that most of us basically have a goal in life to live as long as we can in a state of as good health as possible. I know that is my goal, and it's a goal I've often heard my patients express.

All of us have our own individual reasons in life that motivate us to want to live and enjoy a long, active life. In my case, I realize I'm fortunate to have *many* reasons. Jocelyn and I want to spend more good years together. We have three fine young-adult sons of whom we're very proud—James, Michael, and Andrew. James and Michael have brought into our lives two lovely daughters-in-law, Anne and Laura. We want to watch our sons and their spouses continue to develop and flourish. Also, Jocelyn and I are looking forward to the "grandchildren years" down the road. And, on the professional side, I still have things I want to do as a physician and lecturer—many more things.

Having said that, I know that my weight-loss program increases my chances for enjoying a longer and healthier life.

Think about it: When you go into a senior-living facility that's filled with active seniors, how many 300-pound individuals do you encounter among the residents? Not many. Most people who live the longer, healthier lives are the thinner folks.

It's true that none of us knows what lies around the corner healthwise. But, if we go by statistics and risk factors, I know that by decreasing weight

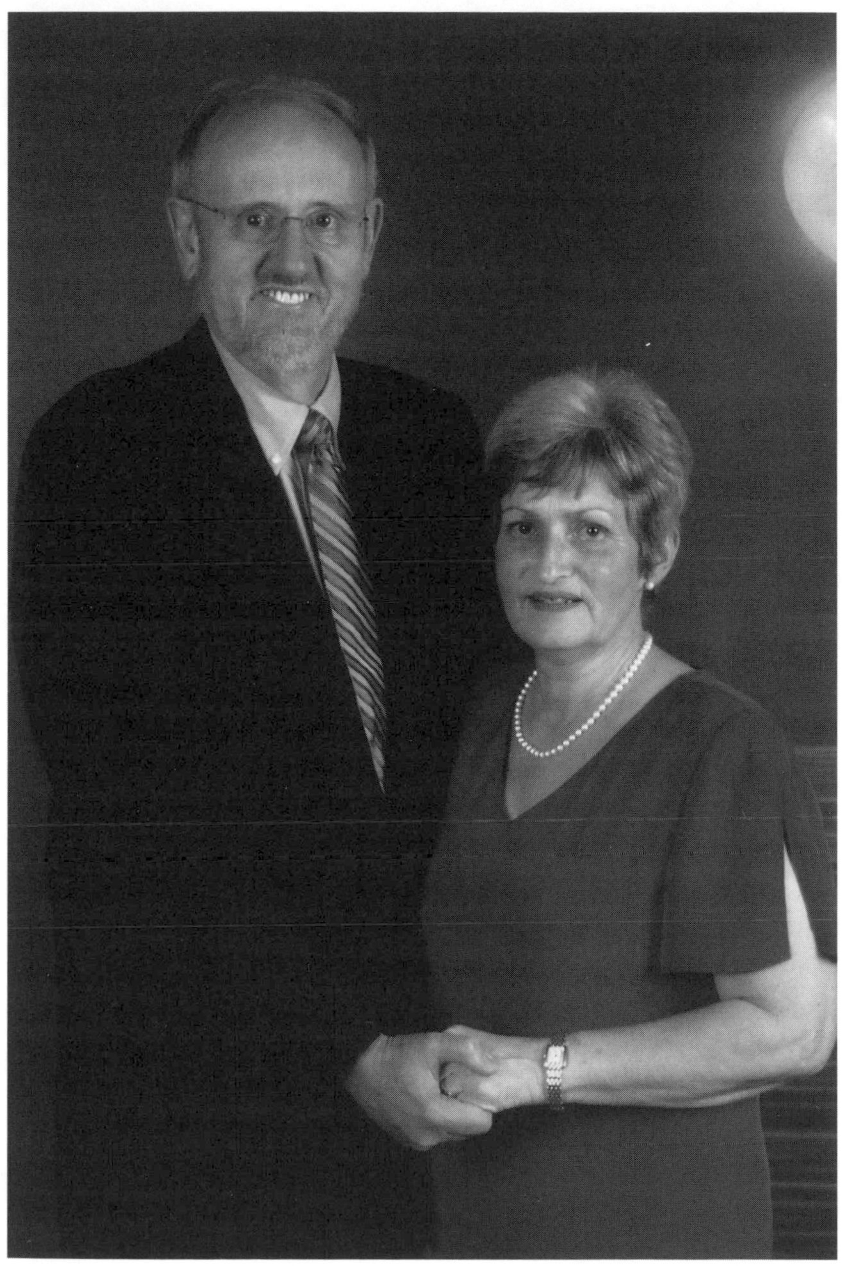

With Jocelyn in late 2004, after I had lost my weight.

and increasing healthy exercise I have reduced, or at least delayed, my own risks in regard to the ravages of overweight-related health problems—problems such as unmanaged high blood pressure, stroke, heart disease, certain cancers, and diabetes.

Note: In Chapters 7–9, I'll give more details about those overweight-related health risk factors.

Feeling Better and Having More Energy

Since I lost this weight, I just *feel* so much better! I had no idea that I could feel this well. I really do believe that if I could have known I would feel this good, I would have been motivated years ago to get this weight off.

One of the main things that makes me feel better is that I have so much more strength, stamina, and energy. Prior to losing weight, I felt fatigued all too often. I would push myself, but still I frequently felt tired and listless.

Even though I'm 64 years old, I find that I'm now able to easily climb stairs and climb hills—things I haven't been able to do perhaps in 20 years! It's a great feeling to be able to manage things I could not manage when I was lugging around all that extra weight.

In terms of how physically active I am these days, my situation is so different and so improved now compared to what it was before my weight loss that it's sometimes difficult for me to comprehend that this is really me.

I'm not talking just about the amount of *programmed* exercise I do. I'm not talking about the time I spend on the treadmill or programmed walking or using the weights. I'm talking about everyday living! If I'm on an outing in which I'm walking around simply for pleasure, I have no problems at all walking for two hours quite rapidly. I have actually done that on occasion and have enjoyed it—enjoyed the process, and also enjoyed the fact I could do it!!

When I go into an office building now, I find that I would rather take the stairs than take the elevator. And, in traveling about doing my medical lecturing, I now enjoy walking in airports rather than my old way of always taking the trains and "people movers" whenever I could.

A Better Night's Sleep for both Jocelyn and Me

As supportive as my wife has been during this weight-loss program, I feel that she should get some benefits out of all this as well.

One clear-cut benefit that has occurred is that I don't snore as much, and therefore Jocelyn and I *both* get more peaceful sleep.

There is no doubt in my mind that this reduction in my snoring is a key reason that I'm not as fatigued. And there is no doubt in my mind that my weight loss caused the reduction in the snoring.

Why is that true? Well, it's a simple fact that when you're obese you are at increased risk to suffer from sleep problems associated with what we call "sleep apnea."

When you have sleep apnea—which I obviously had when I was so obese—several bad things happen:

One is that you tend to snore loudly. Jocelyn said before I lost weight I snored an awful lot.

With sleep apnea, you also tend to have periods when you actually stop breathing for 15 seconds or more and then return to breathing (at least hopefully return to breathing). It's a very quick occurrence in which you stop breathing and then get a "kick" and start breathing again. Jocelyn said that would happen to me during the night as I slept. I also at times was aware it was happening, because I occasionally would wake up with a start when one of those breathing interruptions occurred.

The biggest cause of sleep apnea is obesity. What happens is that when you get overweight there is a tendency for you to collapse your airway. When you lose weight, you aren't as likely to collapse that airway.

Now, as a result of all this snoring and interruption in your breathing as you sleep, obviously you are not getting quality sleep. So another thing that happens is that you often feel tired and fatigued during your "waking hours"—which for me are the more traditional daytime and early evening waking hours.

When you have sleep apnea, you can easily find yourself falling asleep long before your bedtime. That was certainly true in my case. Now, I was going so hard and fast at work seeing patients that I did not have the going-to-sleep problem at work. However, at home in the evening, I could fall asleep at *any* time! All I had to do was to sit down, and I would just nod off to sleep.

All that was happening because I was fat. I'm not fat anymore. So I sleep well, and so does Jocelyn. Also, I don't nod off to sleep during my so-called "waking hours."

Enjoying an Improved Personal Self-Image

All of my life I've tried to downplay in my mind the importance of my personal appearance as it related to my own self-image. I tried to tell myself that it didn't matter to me what other folks thought of how I looked.

Perhaps part of that downplaying related to the fact that I was a fat child, and other children teased me about my weight. I was a strong-willed kid (who grew into a strong-willed adult). So, instead of wilting under the childhood criticism and taunting about my being fat, I rebelled with a defensive attitude of "I don't care anyhow."

Note: I'll have more about this in Chapter 5—that focuses on what it was like to grow up as a fat child.

Now that I'm thin, I would be less than honest with you as the readers of this book if I did not admit that since my weight loss I have been pleased to hear positive comments about my improved appearance. People have told me that I look 10 years younger. I like that, a lot.

I get a charge out of looking in the mirror and knowing within myself that the weight-loss change is good. I can honestly look at myself and say, "You surely do look different!" I enjoy the fact that my clothes fit better (and that the clothes aren't so BIG!)

Of all those who commented positively, none meant more to me than the response from my mother back in my homeland of Northern Ireland. Keep in mind that my mother had known me as an overweight individual most of my life. My mother saw me as a much thinner person when Jocelyn and I paid a visit to Ireland in 2004, after I was deep into my weight-loss program. After giving me an astute visual once-over, my mother said, "David, you look really good!!" I think my mother was really very impressed and quite proud of me. I'll have to tell you that it made me proud to know I had made *her* proud. I'm glad my weight loss (and my keeping it off) occurred during my mother's lifetime. She died in July 2007, at age 88.

Enjoying an Improved Professional Self-Image

My weight loss has really had a positive effect on my self-confidence in two aspects of my medical career.

◊ I feel more self-confident in my role in treating patients.

◊ I feel more self-confident in my role as a medical speaker making clinical presentations to other physicians.

In treating patients, I've never suffered from any lack of self-confidence in my ability to render sound medical care. However, on many an occasion I've had to muster up all my "audacity" to give weight-losing advice to patients when I was not following such advice myself.

I really feel that one of the major benefits my weight loss has brought to me in my professional life is that I'm no longer sitting at a desk advising a patient to lose weight while my gut is hanging over the desk. (In years gone by, I privately referred to my gut as my "Alabama hangover.") You know, it really is very, very difficult to sit there as a severely overweight physician and confidently tell one of your patients, "Now, *you* have got to change *your* lifestyle. *You* have got to lose weight."

Just think about some comparisons: If you were a liver patient and you needed to stop drinking because you had liver damage, how much confidence would you have in a doctor who told you to stop drinking alcohol when the doctor was sitting there talking to you while *he* was reeking of booze? Or, if you were a respiratory patient who really had to stop smoking to protect what was left of your lung capacity, how much confidence would you have in a doctor who is sitting there telling you to stop smoking while *he* smokes a cigarette? It was very much the same thing with my being an overweight doctor telling patients (particularly my patients with diabetes) to drop weight!

In the medical-lecturing part of my career, it has just made me feel much better to be a thin physician standing up there speaking to other physicians in the audiences. All during my overweight years, the topic of my clinical presentations was never diet and exercise itself. The topic was much more likely to be "diabetic heart failure" or some of the newer medications to treat

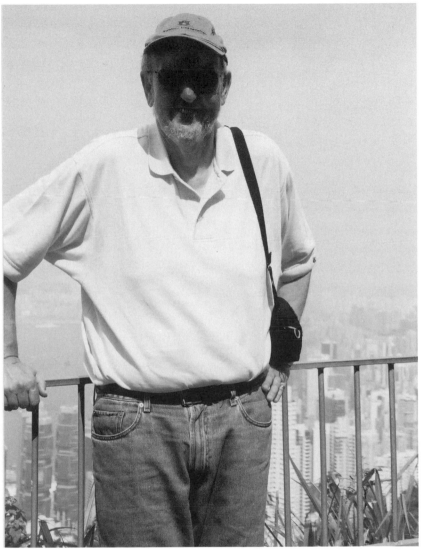

I had shed more than a hundred pounds when this photo was made in Hong Kong in October 2004.

diabetes. Still, even though the topic of my verbal presentations was not diet and exercise, it just makes sense that a thinner, healthier medical lecturer strikes a more credible appearance than a severely overweight one.

I've been pleased with positive responses I've heard from some of the physicians in my audiences concerning my weight loss. And, when a "rumor" got out among some of my colleagues about my weight loss, I really took the rumor as a compliment. The rumor apparently traveled among some of my colleagues who, like myself, are specialists in metabolism. Several of them apparently found it impossible to believe that I was able to lose all this weight "naturally"—that is, to lose it without some type of help.

So the rumor was that I had either undergone gastric bypass surgery or had used some kind of experimental drug. I didn't have the surgery. I didn't take a drug. I simply *pushed back* from the table with my one-meal-a-day plan, and also *pushed forward* with that treadmill, walking, and weight-lifting.

The reason I took this rumor as a compliment is that I think my colleagues were saying, "Hey, man, you have really accomplished something major here!" I liked that.

On May 5, 2007, I participated in (and completed) a 13-mile half-marathon in Indianapolis, Indiana. Consistent with my belief that walking is the best exercise, I walked the half-marathon—finishing in just under 3½ hours, thus averaging about one mile every 16 minutes.

This was fun. I enjoyed a feeling of accomplishment. And, needless to say, this was something I could never have accomplished before I dropped the 100 pounds-plus and got in shape with my exercise regimen.

Getting More Enjoyment Out of Eating!!

Even as I write this book, it amazes me that an increased enjoyment of food ranks high among the benefits I've gotten out of my weight-loss program.

But it's so true!

Since I've lost all this weight and am eating only one meal a day, I am enjoying my food so much more. I eat plenty. I eat what I want. I appreciate food more. I don't have the downside of that uncomfortable feeling I got in the past when I overate and felt so stuffed.

Speaking as the adult version of that fat kid who grew up in Ireland, I can honestly tell you that food is more pleasurable to me than it has been at any time in my entire life!

Part II

Where Did the Obese Person in Me Come From?

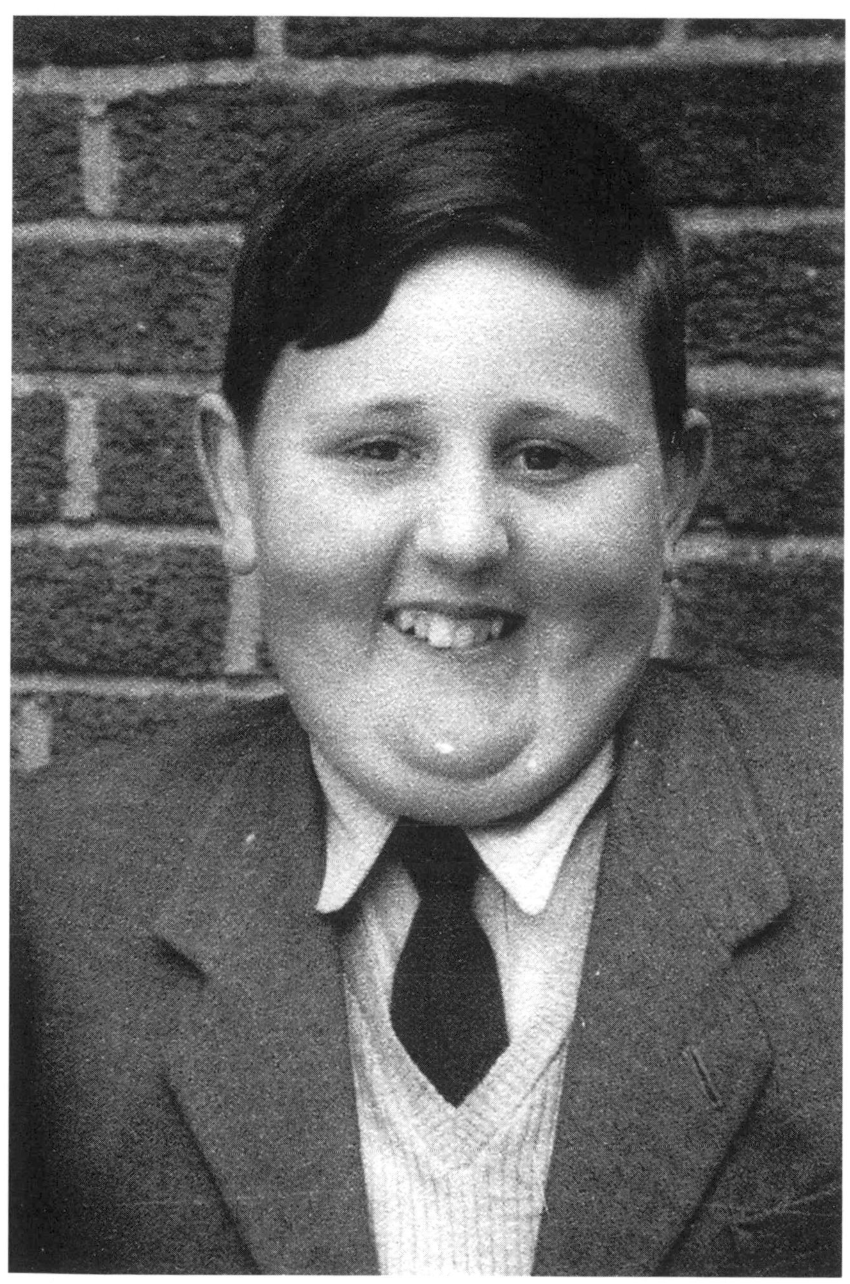

At age 9, I was an overweight child growing up in Northern Ireland.

Chapter 5

YOUNG "BREADAHOLIC"

I came into the world as a fat baby, weighing in at more than 10 pounds. I grew into a fat child. And from there I ate my way into adulthood as a fat adult. My main "tool" in accomplishing this unhealthy feat was BREAD!

Irish Bread "Feeds" a Growing Addiction

Beginning in childhood, I started developing into what I think might well be termed a "breadaholic." Although I over-indulged in eating many types of food, my very favorite indulgence was bread. And bread is not really good for you.

In order for you to understand my love for bread, you must realize that as a child growing up in Ireland, I had access to *very, very nice* breads—exceptionally *delicious* breads.

While some people might think of bread as boring, in Ireland there are many reasons not to think of bread as boring. The Irish have all sorts of great breads. Irish breads are wonderful, and we had all these nice bakeries where we could get all that stuff!

There were so many kinds of tasty breads from which to choose. I loved the breads we call "crumpets"—kind of like pancakes, only smaller and lighter. Then there was "soda bread," which is a whiter bread. I liked "potato bread." I *really* liked a roughly milled, very high-fiber bread called "wheaten bread."

Also, there were so many enjoyable ways to consume the breads. I enjoyed bread with cheese, bread with bananas, bread all by itself. Fried bread was great!

To this day, if I would choose to do so—which I no longer do—I could binge unbelievably on bread.

Other Unhealthy Foods Also on List

Although my very favorite food was bread, I developed a taste for other unhealthy foods as well.

You probably can guess two other fattening, unhealthy types of food that I loved. Fried foods? Yes! Sweets? Yes again!

Among the Irish, I certainly was not alone in my unhealthy food tastes. I look back on my growing-up years in my Northern Ireland homeland and am very aware of how much fried food I saw being consumed—especially fried eggs and fried bacon.

No doubt partly due to that high fat intake, Northern Ireland has laid claim to one of the highest rates of coronary artery disease in the world.

Family Member with the Weight Problem

There were five people in the household in which I was reared—my mother and father, my sister Margaret, 3½ years younger than I; and brother Allan, 8 years younger than I.

I was by far the heaviest eater of the five. And I was the one with a pronounced weight problem.

While my mother tended to carry perhaps 15 pounds more than the "charts" would consider ideal and could have been termed "pleasantly plump," she did not really have a severe weight problem. As for my father, he was very thin, which tended to be a trend on his side of the family.

Both my younger siblings were thin as children, and they became slim adults. There's no question that they ate less than I did. And they tended to seek out healthier, less fattening foods than I did. They ate less bread and were fonder than I was of healthy foods such as cooked vegetables.

"Leave Him Alone"

The undesirable eating patterns I developed and practiced as a child were quite visible for all to see. I was not a "closet eater." When I ate, which was often and a lot, I ate in plain view.

It was clear that I liked to eat and that I focused on eating way too much, that I ate excessively, that I consumed large amounts of food, and that I absolutely tended to eat the wrong kinds of food.

I think parents can be torn about how to handle a child like that. My mother and my father had different ideas. My father won out.

After I reached adulthood and from time to time expressed concern about my weight, my mother often told me that she tried to curtail my calorie intake as I was growing up. However, she said my father told her, "Leave him alone." My father obviously did not want me to be harassed about my eating.

Teasing from Peers

Although I was not harassed at home about over-eating, I was harassed by my childhood peers about being fat.

I was the fattest kid among my childhood peers. I mean, I really was quite overweight, pretty fat. And the contrast stood out, because there weren't that many obese kids back then, in the 1950s.

Unlike the trend today for so many children to be overweight, when I was growing up the trend was for kids to be skinny. The kids who were my childhood neighbors and classmates tended to be skinny.

And, since I was "Fat Boy," that meant that I really did take the teasing!

You know how direct and often unkind children can be to one another. When I was a child, other children called me by the names of famous fat people. Sometimes they called me Fatty Arbuckle—for a popular, and very overweight, American movie actor/comedian. At other times they would call me Churchill—for the legendary, and very rotund—prime minister of Great Britain. There were other names as well that I can't recall. Maybe one reason I can't recall them is kind of "Freudian"—some mind games I played with myself to avoid letting the kids get to me so badly. I tried to switch off their comments.

Although I tried to pretend the teasing didn't matter, I guess it did. I can remember at least one fistfight. I became very angry and emotional because one of my childhood peers said something derogatory about my weight. The kid poked fun at me, and I took a poke at him—with my fists.

A Teacher Shares a Word of Caution

My weight problem was enough of an issue that one of my teachers took it upon herself to try to counsel me about it.

To this day I well remember the concern displayed by that teacher—a lady who was my high school biology teacher. She talked to me very seriously about my overweight condition and its implications. She said, "David, you are far too heavy. You are going to hurt your health. You really need to lose weight."

Exercise in My Youth

Unlike so many fat kids in today's society, at least I did get some exercise during my growing-up years. Keep in mind that I grew up in an era when it was more common for kids to enjoy outdoor playing, that involved running and other physical exertion. That was before today's era when so many kids tend to spend hour after hour in front of televisions, computers, and/or video-games—often while drinking sugar-filled beverages and consuming hamburgers, French fries, and pizza.

One of the outdoor sports I played in my youth was rugby. I played rugby pretty much through high school and for five or six years after high school. However, I cannot tell you that I ever played rugby at a very high level. I didn't play very well at anything, because I was very overweight.

A Class Clown with a Poor Self-Image

There is absolutely no question that being overweight can affect a child's image of himself and can affect his behavior and personality.

Regardless of whether the child admits it or not—and I tended not to admit it—a child tends to reacts strongly to peer criticism and ridicule.

My own reaction to being teased and taunted about being a fat child was that I often tried to be everybody's friend. The way I did that was to be funny, to make my friends laugh. I became the class clown much of the way through my school years.

It wasn't until later in life that I realized all this teasing helped me form a poor self-image as it related to my body image. I guess I was fortunate that I was a goal-oriented kid, and that I was achieving in other ways—including academics and going on to college and into a profession, as a physician, that I enjoyed. So I can't say that as I grew from childhood into adulthood I felt totally insecure or totally unfulfilled. I was pretty much okay with other areas of my life, except for the way I viewed my appearance much of the time.

But a poor body self-image is not something to be dismissed, and in my case there is no doubt it was directly related to my childhood obesity.

Starting the Up-and-Down Weight Cycle

If a child enters his teenage years in a state of obesity, that can be particularly devastating. Girls enter the equation, and if you're an obese person you won't tend to be as popular with the girls as you would if you were thinner. And it's not just with the girls. As a fat kid, you don't tend to be as popular *period* as you would if you were thin.

While I still was in high school, I finally became concerned enough about my weight to shed some pounds. I started losing the weight at a point when I was at around 260 pounds—a pretty hefty teenager. By the time I graduated from high school I was down to 215 pounds, almost as thin as I am now.

But that was not to last. As a medical student, my weight would soar, up to the 300-pound range.

It was a part of an up-and-down weight cycle (much more *up* than down) that I would continue on for decades, until I would devise and use the One-Plus-One Weight-Loss Plan.

Chapter 6

Tackling Life's Challenges—Except Being Overweight

It is my view that one of the most difficult things you can do in life is to tackle the problem of being overweight, particularly if you're *severely* overweight.

That's why I say so often, "Losing weight is *not* for wimps."

I certainly don't think that all overweight individuals are weak, indecisive people. I mean, why would I think THAT? I don't think I'm a weak person. And my track record is not that of being an indecisive person. I was just, for a long time, a *fat* person.

This weight thing is just plain difficult, in many ways.

There's a lot of *self-indulgence* mixed in with eating. We eat for a lot of reasons besides being hungry.

There's a lot of pure *habit* mixed in with eating.

There is certainly a lot of *temptation* mixed in with eating. For those of us fortunate enough to live in civilized, affluent societies, we have food around us all the time—too much food.

Too, maybe above all, there is a lot of *denial* mixed in with eating. There is denial on two major fronts. First of all, sometimes we tend to deny we are overweight even when we know we're overweight. And secondly, even if we admit we're overweight we tend to deny that being overweight is *really* a problem—namely a problem associated with health risks. We often tend to deny that being fat is a problem until the poor-health consequences are staring us in the face, such as with my own skyrocketing blood pressure. (And, as I have noted before and will note again, because it's well worth noting: Many people aren't lucky enough to get a warning. Many overweight people suffer major health problems before they do anything about their weight. Some people die of weight-related health problems before they get a chance to do anything about their weight.)

Prior to my decision to lose weight, I experienced all of the issues I've just mentioned. I experienced self-indulgence, habit, temptation, and denial.

A Personal Journey

In this chapter I want to take you on a very personal journey through three major challenges I faced when I was in my 20s. These were situations in which I had to made decisions that had far-reaching impact on my life. In each of the three cases, the decisions were tough.

I look back on those decisions now and sometimes question why I was able to confront those three particular challenges but at the same time I was not able (or not willing) to confront my weight problem in a lasting way.

My Reasons for this Chapter

I think that all too often when someone writes a weight-loss book that the author tends to preach rather than teach, that he or she tends to despair rather than to share and care, that he or she tends to vilify other people rather than identify with other people.

Let me be the first to tell you that if you are fat and you don't want to be fat but you have not been able to lose weight and keep it off, I can identify with you. I was that way a long time. And I'll have to keep up the good fight (keep my weight off), or I'll be back in that situation again.

I do feel that I have some internal strengths that I could have harnessed years ago to tackle my own weight issue. Many of you reading this book likely have some internal strengths you could harness in dealing with your own weight problem. Perhaps, through reading this book, something will trigger inside of you that will help you with some positive "harnessing."

What I'm saying is simply this: If you have been able to tackle one kind of challenge in your own life, why not use that strength to tackle the being-overweight challenge?

Through this chapter, I hope you'll understand a little more about *me.*

At the same time through this chapter I hope you'll understand a little more about *you.*

As you read the next few pages, you'll see the inside of my own experiences in which I had to look myself in the mirror and say, "Hey, David, this situation is not working the way it stands now. You've got to find a better way."

Time and again, I was able to find a better way. Yet, even as I had these experiences, I was a fat guy who deep down inside knew that being so fat *also* was a situation that was not working for me. Where my weight was concerned, I went decades before I sought and found a better way to lose weight and keep it off.

As you read about me in these following pages, I invite you to also think about yourself and what makes *you* tick.

Just as I have had challenging situations that I did something about, you have had difficult situations in *your own life.* If you're overweight, and you have handled other situations but not your weight, maybe you could let your thoughts travel to the "why" behind that as well.

My Three "Turning-Point" Situations

◊ I changed career goals in mid-stream, after investing a lot of time and study in my first career goal.

◊ I made a decision to stop smoking cigarettes.

◊ After much soul-searching, I left my native country and family and friends I loved because I felt it was just not the place for me to be at that time.

Trading Dentistry for Medicine

When I was completing my pre-college studies at the Belfast Royal Academy in Northern Ireland, I settled on the career path I would pursue. I chose clinical dentistry.

I saw dentistry as a profession I would enjoy, one that I would find rewarding, and one that would produce a good living. Too, several of my peers—young people in my age group whom I respected—were planning to enroll or had already enrolled in dental school. In those days, dentists in the United Kingdom generally were doing quite well financially, and to me it seemed a good direction to take.

But, even though dentistry seemed a "match" for me at the time, over the next few years I would discover something about myself that concerned me as it related to clinical dentistry.

As I pursued my studies in clinical dentistry at Queens University/Belfast Dental School between 1962 and 1965, I had to struggle somewhat with a part of dentistry that was quite central to the profession—manual dexterity. The further I moved along in my dental studies, and the more that was demanded of me in the way of manual dexterity, the more I realized my manual skills were not what I felt they needed to be.

It took awhile for me to really confront this situation. By the time I did confront it, I was halfway into the fourth year of a five-year course in clinical dentistry. As I "dissected" this situation, I looked at some realities head-on: Yes, I could complete dental school. But no, I did not think I would actually hang out my shingle as a practicing dentist. If I completed my dental education, I more likely would go into teaching dentistry or into some avenue of dental research. To me, that would mean I would be participating in only part of the dental profession. I knew that I would not be satisfied with placing those kinds of limitations on my career.

So, even though I already was quite far down the road in my dental studies, I made the decision to look seriously in another career direction.

During my years in dental school, I had been exposed to hospital medicine. I had developed a strong liking for what I had observed in my glimpses into the world of medicine. Pursuing a career as a physician held appeal to me. So I applied to medical school at the much-respected Queens University School of Medicine, and I got in! I felt very lucky.

That decision to become a physician led me into the fruitful decades I've enjoyed so much as a specialist in internal medicine and subspecialist in endocrinology and diabetes and metabolism. During these productive decades, I've never once looked back and felt that I "wasted" those three and a half years in dental education. Quite the contrary. I believe those years of dental education further strengthened my education as a physician.

However, I do look back now and realize that changing career objectives in mid-stream was a pretty big "changing-gears" decision for a young man in his 20s to be making. I'm proud I made that decision. I knew I had a problem, and I thought it out and changed course.

During that period in my life, why couldn't I have been that proactive in taking action to keep my weight under control?

Cigarettes Become the Enemy

Back in my high school days, it seemed to be the "cool thing to do" for many of the kids to sneak around and smoke two or three cigarettes after school. I was one of those kids. We knew we weren't supposed to be smoking cigarettes. Knowing that cigarette smoking was forbidden was no doubt part of the reason *we did it anyhow.* As kids, we actually were drawn to the fact that smoking cigarettes was taboo. That made it all that much more fun. If our elders had told us it was okay to do it, we probably would not have tried it.

As all too many folks know, this sneaking of a cigarette here and there easily can lead to regular cigarette smoking. The first thing you know, you are addicted to cigarettes. In many people, cigarette smoking is a very severe addiction, perhaps more addictive than narcotics.

By the time I was first a dental student and then a medical student, I was smoking cigarettes regularly.

Then, very abruptly, my days of cigarette smoking came to an end. To me, cigarettes became the enemy. For cigarettes claimed the life of someone I loved very much—my father.

My father was 61 years of age when he was diagnosed with lung cancer. He didn't last long after the diagnosis. He never made it to age 62.

Since my father was a cigarette smoker, I didn't have to go far to add two plus two and get four. Research already had linked cigarette smoking to lung cancer and a host of other health problems.

In my view, cigarettes became the enemy. The last day I ever smoked a cigarette was the day my father was diagnosed with lung cancer. I was 28 years old.

I made a positive decision in the midst of a terribly negative situation. My putting down cigarettes was partly a reaction to my bereavement about my father. It also was a recognition that cigarettes had done bad things to my father. I wanted to prevent that from happening to me as well.

However, at the same time I was walking away from my addiction to cigarette smoking I still was in the grips of my addiction to overeating.

Feeling Insecure in a Beloved Homeland

The further along I got into my medical training, the more convinced I became that I had made the right choice when I decided to become a physician.

My professional life was especially good in the early 1970s, when I was an intern and then a resident in the prestigious, rich-in-heritage Royal Victoria Hospital in Belfast, Northern Ireland—quite a famous hospital. Learning and working at Royal Victoria was an incredible experience.

There also were some happy developments in my personal life. During my first rotation as an intern at Royal Victoria—a rotation in neurosurgery—I met Jocelyn Johnston, a young staff nurse from Southern Ireland. Jocelyn and I began a 15-month courtship that culminated in our marriage in November 1971. After our marriage, Jocelyn and I settled in an apartment near the hospital, where I continued my residency and Jocelyn continued to work as a nurse.

There were so many positive things about that period. Life could have been great then. However, there was one massive overriding and ongoing crisis spreading a dark cloud that neither Jocelyn nor I could control. By living in Northern Ireland, and especially by living in Belfast, we were living in a principal battleground for an ongoing civil war.

As you will recall from your history, this civil war in Northern Ireland was known as The Troubles. The conflict was waged from the late 1960s on forward for some 35 years. Some of the worst of the violence that would erupt over the decades in war-ravaged Belfast came during the early 1970s—including Bloody Sunday and Bloody Friday, both in 1972.

It was a civil war that pitted Protestants against Catholics, that pitted the Unionists' community against the Nationalists' community, that staked out bitter conflicting views as to the degree of independence Northern Ireland should or should not have from Great Britain.

These differences of opinion were played out with gunfire and bombs, with thousands of injuries and fatalities in and around Belfast alone, in addition to victims in other areas in Northern Ireland.

As Jocelyn and I tried to build and maintain a meaningful existence in our homeland during these difficult times, we found ourselves ministering to victims of violence in our roles as nurse and physician. Also, there were occasions in which we came all too close to becoming victims of violence ourselves.

I recall one troubling incident after another that ultimately would lead to our pivotal life-changing decision to leave our homeland.

I remember, for example, working as a physician in the emergency room at Royal Victoria Hospital the day they brought in a young man in his early 20s who had been shot in the neck. Now, this boy himself had taken no part in anything political. Instead, he had been shot because of who his father was. His father was a member of the official IRA (Irish Republican Army), and the boy had been shot by another faction of the IRA. The image of this young man is still firmly implanted in my mind even today. As soon as I got to him when he came into the ER, I saw the bullet wound to his neck. I began to assess him quickly. His vital signs were fine. I told him, "You're fine. You're fine. Your blood pressure is fine. You're doing okay. You haven't bled much." And he looked up at me and asked, "Then why can't I move my f---ing arms and legs???!!!" They had shot him straight through the spine. That kid was left a quadriplegic—paralyzed from the neck down, for the rest of his shortened life. Not because of anything he had done. But just because of who he was—actually, because of who his father was.

Then there were the chilling experiences I encountered in gunfire-ridden Belfast as I went out into communities to make house calls. This was not my regular hospital job. This was my "moonlighting" job. A lot of young resident-physicians did moonlighting, in which we would go out at night and handle home-based medical care for general practitioners. This moonlighting was set up to be a win-win-win system for everyone involved: It gave overworked general practitioners some time at home with their families at night, and made it possible for them to get some much-needed sleep; it provided an extra layer of night-time medical services for people in the community; and it rewarded young physicians such as myself with additional patient-care experience and some extra cash to help make ends meet.

Well, obviously when you venture out to take care of patients in their homes, you go wherever the sick folks live. In Belfast in the 1970s, some of those sick folks were living in very dangerous neighborhoods where people were shooting at one another. As I tried to make my way to the homes of individuals who had called for medical help, often I found it difficult to even see where I was going, because the people doing battle in the streets had shot out all the lights and removed all the street signs.

One night I had just come out of an apartment building where I had made a house call to a patient. I was on my way to my car. And all of a sudden a bullet came zooming past my head. I wasn't hit. I was just scared half out of my wits. As I look back, the car I was driving could easily have looked like a police car at night in that bleak darkness. I don't think they were shooting *at* me. I mean, I don't think I was actually the target. But the bullet certainly came *toward* me.

On another occasion I was called to the home of a woman who was in the throes of a life-threatening asthma attack. When I reached her neighborhood, there was a riot going on. This group of angry people approached my car and tried to stop me from going into the area. I said, "I've got to go in there. There's a woman with asthma. I need to get in." One of the rioters who was trying to stop me, an older man, said to me, "Let her die!" I told him, "No, I'm not going to do that. I've got to get in." Finally they let me pass. I drove to where the woman lived, was able to help her medically, and made it back to my home in one piece.

On still another occasion, I had to get past a group of rioting children who were throwing stones. These young children were actually being supervised in their violence by a woman. This woman came over and talked to me, I told her my business as a doctor, and she authorized the kids to stop throwing the stones and let me pass on through.

One very disturbing experience I encountered had to do with dangerous information about a violent incident that a patient started to tell me before I stopped her. It was information about a man who recently had been murdered by one of the warring factions there in Belfast. The patient who started to tell me this information was a woman who lived in an apartment-housing development where I was doing some "moonlighting" work in a doctor's office. The woman came to this little doctor's office and proceeded to tell me that she was so nervous and distraught that I just had to write her a prescription for a strong tranquilizer to calm her nerves. Well, I don't believe in just writing prescriptions without first finding out details about a patient's situation. So I asked her, "What is your problem? Why would you need a medication so strong to calm your nerves?" When she began to tell me, I could see why she was so upset. This woman was in terror! She told me that she actually had witnessed some people take the murder victim away from this particular apartment building shortly before he was murdered. I stopped her cold, before she could tell me more. That information was not something I should be hearing. This was just information that I did not need! To tell the truth, I don't know who, if anyone, this woman should have been telling this to during those treacherous, troubled times in Northern Ireland. Based on what I had seen, if she had reported what she saw, nothing would have been done about it. She would have just put herself in jeopardy. I felt, too, that if I listened further I would be in jeopardy as well. Although I had asked her to tell me what was troubling her, I felt it was in her best interest and mine as well to stop her from going further. I can still recall how stunned I was sitting in that office talking to this poor woman, and hoping that the wrong people weren't listening through the paper-thin walls of that building! There was just an intimidating, violent atmosphere all around.

The violence that spread through Northern Ireland during that period was affecting my own family members as well. My sister's husband was kidnapped. My sister was held up by terrorists in the bank where she worked, during a bank robbery. I had a police-sergeant uncle who learned he was on a terrorist "hit list." My uncle could not even visit my dying father in the hospital, because the hospital was located in an area of Belfast that was heavily populated by that terrorist group. My police-sergeant uncle had a son (my first cousin) who also was a police officer. One day while this cousin of mine was on police duty near a school, a group of terrorists drove by in a car and fired on him with a machine gun. Amazingly, he survived even though he was sprayed *with a total of 24 bullets*—22 of the bullets hitting his flak jacket (bulletproof vest), and the other two claiming the vision in one of his eyes and destroying the hearing in one of his ears.

Then came the terrifying incident that turned out to be the clincher for Jocelyn and me. It occurred in September 1972. Jocelyn and I had been married for 10 months. We had just been on vacation to Rumania. Although our vacation itself was mostly enjoyable, at the end of our holiday we experienced an extremely tense airplane flight home from Rumania. The flight was a delayed, bumpy, horrendous airplane ride on a Russian-made prop jet—a type of jet that in the coming months would be associated with a number of crashes. After Jocelyn and I miraculously made it home safely to Belfast following that harrowing flight, we focused on relaxing. Our goal was to enjoy a bit of peace and quiet before it was time for us to return to work at the hospital. Sadly, that was not to be. We had been home only a few hours when we heard the sounds of gunfire outside our little apartment. When the shots were fired, Jocelyn was standing in the kitchen, preparing our evening meal. I ushered her into the bedroom, which at least did not have a wall to the outside. (Although, looking back, I realize those walls were so vulnerable that the bullets could easily have made their way to the bedroom if they had been headed in that direction.) A few minutes later, after the gunfire ceased, Jocelyn and I discovered that one of the bullets had come through the kitchen window of our apartment. The bullet had lodged in a cabinet very near where Jocelyn had been standing as she prepared our dinner—in fact, in a spot that was just above Jocelyn's head!! Jocelyn and I never spent another night in that apartment. We evacuated.

That did it! Although Jocelyn and I had been born and reared in Ireland, she in the South and I in the North, we both talked it over and said, "Maybe there's a message here. Maybe we're being told something." We decided we were leaving. It became a choice of going to Africa or going to Canada. I was encouraged by my mentors not to go to Africa, because a very unstable situation existed there as well. So we went to Canada, and several years later we would move again, to relocate in the United States.

In one sense, one might say it's a "no-brainer" to make a decision to leave a situation such as the one I described in Northern Ireland in the early 1970s. And in a sense that's true. Jocelyn and I both agreed it was time to leave. We were in a war-torn country, and we didn't see a future for ourselves there. It would prove to be a good decision to go to Canada for me to practice medicine and Jocelyn to work as a nurse and registered nurse-midwife. A few years later, it would be another good decision for us to move on from Canada to the United States.

At the same time, it's not easy to leave behind your roots, your family, friends you've had all your life. Those relationships you form in your early years are special, unique, never to be replaced in exactly the same way.

When I left Northern Ireland, I departed not just with the memories of the sectarian and political violence. I departed also with some vivid, wonderful childhood memories of a country so rich in history and heritage and legends, a country that could be unbelievably beautiful and inviting when not torn apart with bombs and gunfire. I left with warm memories of the Irish town of Armagh in which I lived until we moved to Belfast when I was age 8, memories of so many very enjoyable times in Belfast, and memories of hanging out with the farm animals and gathering eggs on my uncle's farm in the little community of Mackerknock near Belfast. I left with images of watching the salmon jump in the Bush River. This is that same river that flows near the oldest licensed whiskey distillery in the world, Old Bushmills Distillery—with its first permit dating back to the 17th century and its roots probably three centuries prior to that. I left with memories of feeling like such a strong kid the first time I swam all the way across a bay near the legendary Giant's Causeway tourist attraction on the northeastern coast of Northern Ireland, near Scotland. Oh, how impressed I was with this Giant's Causeway that some have called the "eighth wonder of the world," with its unique hexagon-shaped rocks and its legend of having been the long-ago chosen battleground of Irish giant Finn McCool and his Scottish adversary Benandonner. I left Northern Ireland also with memories of the pride that swelled inside me when good things came my way. I recall, for instance, how proud I felt as I lined up for drill competition with the Boys Brigade (kind of like the Boy Scouts). And I left with the memory of accomplishment when I learned in grade six that I had just passed a door-opening examination—an exam that guaranteed me a slot in a high school that could prepare me for the higher level of education I sought.

So, when Jocelyn and I left Northern Ireland in 1973, the memories I held certainly included a lot of good. Although I knew it was time to go, the decision to leave was one of the most poignant, and certainly one of the most far-reaching, in my life.

Change after Change

So it was that much of my life in my 20s and on into my 30s was like a fast-moving slide show, flashing from change to more change.

Among circumstances that changed during that period was my weight. It went *down*. I got down to a pretty decent, normal size while I was in Canada. For a while, I kind of had this weight thing under control.

Looking back, one has to wonder if some of that weight loss wasn't connected with heavy, heavy stress, punctuated by major, major, change.

Whatever the reason, I didn't stay slim over the long haul. A few years later, when Jocelyn and I relocated to the southern part of the United States, I was told by several friends:

"David, down south they have good food and a lot of it."

"Much of Southerners' socializing revolves around food."

"People in the southern United States tend to use a lot of fat in cooking their food."

"David, you had better watch it after you move south, or you could really put on a great deal of weight."

Their warnings and predictions proved to be all too true.

Part III

Your Loved Ones and Your Weight

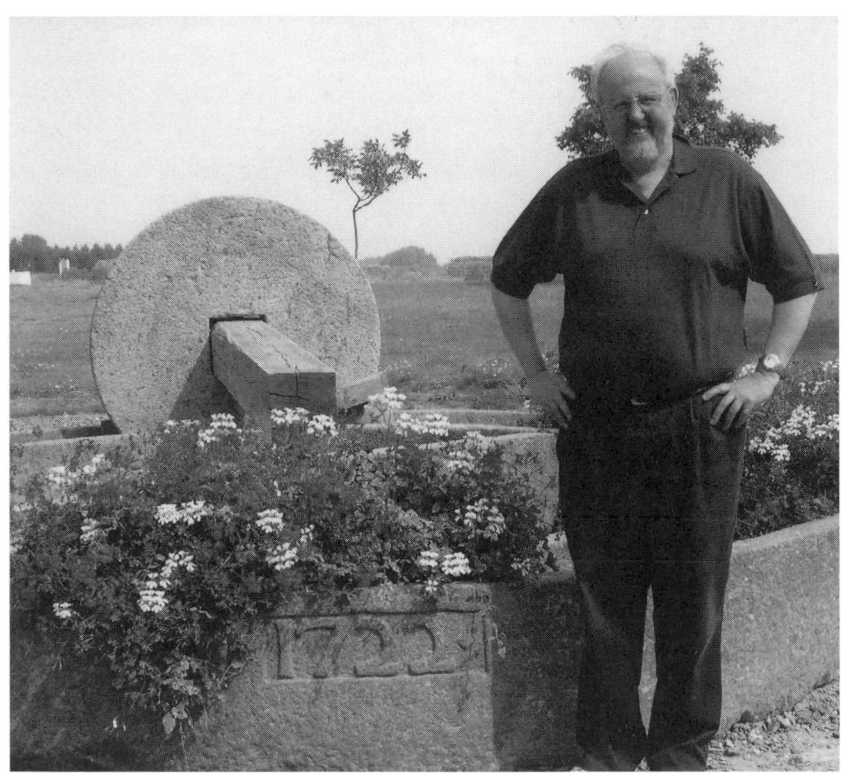

This photo was taken in France about the time I launched my weight-loss program in the summer of 2003. Up to this time, I had not accepted that being overweight was a big problem for me.

Chapter 7

Understanding the Risks of Being Overweight

Whenever you come face-to-face with a problem, you have a better chance of licking it if you *understand* it.

Being overweight definitely qualifies as being a problem. Suffice it to say that being much *too big* is a *big* problem. It's a problem not only in terms of how you look—your vanity issues. It's also a big problem in terms of your health—putting you at risk to suffer major health problems and perhaps die prematurely.

I've already admitted to you that it has only been since 2003 that I have *really* accepted the truths about being overweight as those truths apply to me.

It was terribly difficult for me to face that my overweight condition was placing me in jeopardy. I was stubborn about applying those realities to myself even though I had decades of experience as a physician. I was stubborn even though I am a physician who specializes in the field of endocrinology, metabolism, and diabetes—areas in which weight control is a major issue.

When my high-blood-pressure crisis finally forced me to confront some truths, I looked at information about excessive weight gain from a whole new perspective—a very personal perspective. I revisited huge amounts of weight-related data I had encountered as a physician. Then I added many personal insights I acquired as being someone whose weight reached well over 300 pounds (probably around 325)!

I believe my professional exposure and my very personal journey in weight control have equipped me to advise you, the reader, about key bits of information you need to know if you really are going to understand excessive weight gain and its risks.

What Do You Need to Know?

What do you need to know in order to understand the implications of being significantly overweight?

You need to know the extent of the "being-overweight" epidemic.

You need to understand the risks associated with being overweight.

And you need to know why so many people are overweight these days—that is, what it is about our society that's making so many people so fat.

If you or one of your loved ones is among the large numbers of overweight people, I hope you learn something in this book that helps you (or them) to separate yourselves from society's dangerous overweight trends.

The Extent of the "Being-Overweight" Epidemic

Increasing numbers of people in many developed nations around the globe are falling into the categories of being either "overweight" or "obese." As you know, being "obese" is just a fatter version of being "overweight."

In the United States, the main governmental agency that tracks excessive weight gain and the resulting problems is the Centers for Disease Control and Prevention, (CDC), a part of the U.S. Department of Health and Human Services. In recent years, the CDC time and again has issued alarming reports about the rising numbers of people who are overweight or obese.

According to the CDC, an estimated 65 percent of U.S. adults aged 20 years and older are either overweight or obese.

In recent years, federal officials in the United States have become so alarmed about citizens' excessive weight gain that one report after another has been issued to try to motivate overweight people to lose weight. A key example of these reports is *The Surgeon General's Call to Action to Prevent and Decrease Overweight and Obesity; What Can You Do?*

These are indications of concern from just one major developed nation, the United States. From my own perspective, I can tell you that this increasing incidence of excessive weight doesn't just exist in the United States. This problem is widespread in developed nations all over the world!

Fatter Children

As parents, we sometimes like to joke and say, "Don't do as I *do*. Do as I *say*!" Well, maybe it's not always a joke when we say it.

In the area of gaining too much weight, there's no doubt that children are emulating their parents. If we as adults don't control our own weight, how can we expect our children to control theirs?

In looking at today's children as a group, we can see they are getting fatter and fatter. Many children are doing the same thing their parents are doing. They are eating too much, taking in too many calories and too much fat. And, of equal importance, they are exercising too little.

If you are a parent in your 30s, 40s, 50s, or 60s, you likely can recall going through school with a classroom of relatively thin classmates. By way of contrast, look at the children in today's school classrooms. Today's classrooms are full of overweight children!

This frightening statistic from the Centers for Disease Control and Prevention tells the story: *In the United States today, an estimated 16 percent of children and adolescents ages 6-19 are overweight. That means that one out of every six children in this nation is listed by the CDC as being overweight!* Compared to 20 years ago, that's nearly double the rate of overweight or obese conditions among the nation's children.

Federal health officials are extremely concerned. One focus among recent CDC reports on weight gain in the U.S. is entitled: *The Surgeon General's Call to Action to Prevent and Decrease Overweight and Obesity; Overweight in Children and Adolescents.*

There is no doubt that this alarming weight gain among children is doing a great disservice to children in terms of their health. If you look just at this one statistic alone, it's enough to send chills up your spine: *You must realize that one in every three children born in this country today will develop diabetes. And if the child is in a high-risk minority group, that statistic rises to one out of every two who will develop diabetes!* The chief overriding factor that's contributing to this rise in diabetes among children is the rising incidence of excessive weight in children.

On top of the diabetes risk, overweight children are likely to grow up to be overweight adults—overweight adults who face the serious adult health risks that excessive weight brings.

Those health risks are many. And they are frightening. Here's an overview:

Health Risks of Being Too Fat

I don't know one good thing that being overweight or obese can do for your health!

Quite the contrary.

Every major modern-day disease and unhealthy condition we can think of is made worse in some way, or ways, by excessive weight.

If you are an adult who is significantly overweight, you are more likely to get these diseases or conditions, you are less likely to be diagnosed promptly and accurately, or you are less likely to respond well to treatment—or all three.

Because so many people are so fat, we see the following:

◊ There is more lung disease.

◊ There's more heart disease—ranging from coronary artery disease, to heart attacks, to other heart problems as well.

◊ There's more high blood pressure, more strokes.

◊ There's more stomach disease.

◊ There's more reflux of acid into the esophagus.

◊ There's more sleep apnea—periods in which breathing ceases during sleep. Sleep apnea clearly is a condition that tends to be associated with obesity. The people who have sleep apnea also tend to have more heart disease, more heart failure, and more strokes.

◊ There's more arthritis, more joint damage. If you are carrying too much weight, arthritis can become a *real* problem to you.

◊ There's more infertility.

◊ There is higher incidence of heavy bleeding from the womb.

◊ Several cancers are associated with obesity. Cancer of the pancreas is one. Cancer of the bowels is another. And obese women are at higher risk to get breast cancer.

◊ Being overweight also puts you at risk for a health problem that many individuals might not know about—called "metabolic syndrome" or "insulin-resistance syndrome." This is a condition in which you have excess fat in the cavity around the organs in your abdomen—the peritoneal cavity. This excess fat produces chemicals that can cause inflammation. That inflammation in turn can set the stage for hardening of the blood vessels (atherosclerosis). You can suffer spasms in the blood vessels. You can experience abnormal clotting. You can increase your risk of heart disease as much as five times the normal rate.

◊ Many, many people in this nation—both children and adults—are developing diabetes partly because they have put on too much weight. The harsh fact is that if you gain excessive amounts of weight, you automatically put yourself at much higher risk to develop Type 2 diabetes.

The Diabetes Risk

I've treated diabetes for a long time. I've seen up-close the horrible toll that diabetes takes in terms of unhealthy lives, amputations, loss of vision, kidney failure, heart problems, and premature death.

Diabetes is a disease associated with function of the body's pancreas.

Diabetes is a disease also linked to genetics—that is, it tends to "run" in families.

Then, too, diabetes is a disease often related to excessive weight. The more obese people become, the more diabetes will occur and the earlier in life the diabetes will tend to occur. (Too, the earlier in life one gets diabetes, the more complications one is likely to suffer.)

If you have a family history of diabetes, and if you have a susceptible pancreas, and you gain excessive amounts of weight, then you are *really* at risk for developing diabetes.

Let's say you put on a good bit of weight and you are evaluating your chances of developing diabetes as a result. One big factor is how strong your pancreas is to begin with.

So…let's compare your chances to something many of us know about—cars. Assume that you start out with a luxury-car pancreas—a real high-quality, top-of-the line pancreas. And let's assume you have no family history of diabetes. Now, if this is true, you just might be able to get fat and never develop diabetes. (However, even if you miss diabetes, that does not put you in the clear. Your excessive weight gain still could put you on the path toward one or more of the other health problems I have just listed.)

But let's say that you start out with a "jalopy" pancreas—an old rundown pancreas that is like a jalopy rundown car. You proceed to put on some weight. Even if you don't have a family history of diabetes, a weight gain of as little as 10 pounds could tilt you over the edge in developing diabetes.

But then most of us fall somewhere in between. We have a pancreas like an ordinary run-of-the-mill automobile—nothing luxurious, but not real rundown. So let's say that you have that kind of middle-of-the-road average pancreas, and you start putting on weight. You're rolling the dice. Your chances of developing diabetes are around 50-50.

Weight Gain and Chronic-Disease Epidemics

As people get fatter, we are steadily increasing our risks of major epidemics of chronic diseases.

I'm referring to chronic diseases such as heart disease, and lung disease, and diabetes, and arthritis.

All of these diseases are tied in one way or another with weight. Being overweight is a major risk factor.

Partly because of the epidemic of excessive weight gain, I firmly believe we are headed for epidemics of chronic diseases. And I believe the first of these that is already rearing its ugly head is the epidemic of diabetes.

Most of these chronic diseases are diseases that tend to go on and on in terms of their duration. People tend to suffer from them for years. Usually these chronic diseases are diseases for which there is no cure, they are diseases that are expensive to treat, and they are diseases that tend to lessen both the quality and the length of their victims' lives.

Epidemics of chronic diseases are crises with which civilized societies have little experience. Up until now, our experience with disease epidemics mainly has been with epidemics of contagious diseases, not chronic diseases.

As we are well aware, chronic diseases are not diseases that we can "catch" from someone else. They are diseases that occur on an individual basis inside a person's body. You don't "catch" chronic diseases such as diabetes or cancer or arthritis.

By contrast, contagious diseases are transmitted first to one human and then another—sometimes directly from person to person; other times with the help of infected animals, birds, and insects; other times with the aid of a contaminated environment.

Probably the most well-known contagious disease epidemic of all time to date has been The Plague, often called "bubonic plague," and also known as Black Death. It was spread to humans by fleas on rats and some species of mice. The Plague was of such proportions it qualified as a "pandemic"—a massive epidemic that cut a wide geographical path and wiped out large percentages of populations. The Plague had its root in the late Middle Ages—in the 1300s—and it killed nearly a third of the population in the British Isles. When The Plague returned with a vengeance in the mid-1600s, the British Isles again were hard hit. The situation was so deplorable that carts were driven through the streets each night to pick up the latest victims who had died that day, with the drivers simply calling in loud voices, "Bring out yer dead!"

Another well-known contagious disease catastrophe was the Great Influenza Epidemic of 1918–1919. This powerful flu spread around the world, wiping out entire villages in some nations, devastating World War I troop units, and all in all killing millions. Even on the low end of estimates, statisticians tell us that this flu "pandemic" claimed at least 25 million lives; other statisticians tell us it was much worse—maybe claiming two to three times that many.

If we just look at the financial aspect, there's a big, big difference in the tab that society paid for the contagious disease epidemics of the past and the money that will be spent on the chronic disease epidemics that are now upon us. Let's take a look at why there is such difference:

Those contagious diseases of the past such as The Plague and the Great Influenza Epidemic without doubt took tremendous emotional tolls beyond our comprehension—emotional tolls associated with loss of life. However, there was not a huge financial toll associated with those contagious diseases of the past. One reason there was a relatively low financial toll is because there were so few effective treatments for these contagious diseases—so little treatment on which to spend money. Too, the diseases didn't tend to hang around very long. Simply stated, those contagious diseases of the past were so lethal that they ran their course quickly; people either got well or they died. Those who survived usually survived with few if any problems. So the cost to the system was not real high.

In grave contrast, with the epidemics of chronic diseases that we now face, the financial toll will be outlandish—probably more than the system can stand. That is already proving to be the case. In this day and age, treatments are available to help manage chronic diseases and their complications; and those treatments cost huge amounts of money. Too, a number of the chronic diseases do tend to hang around for a long time. For example, consider the cost issues associated with diabetes. The cost in treating diabetes is not just with insulin, needles, pills, medicated strips to test the fingersticks, doctors' visits, and laboratory costs. *The real cost of diabetes is the treatment of complications of diabetes*—kidney dialysis, kidney transplants, expensive treatment in intensive care units, coronary artery bypass grafts, management of stroke victims, long-term care for debilitated patients with diabetes, and on and on.

The reason I go into detail about this is that if we don't get a handle on some of our chronic diseases—like diabetes and heart disease and various cancers—we are going to see unfathomable epidemics of chronic diseases, the like of which the world has never seen! These epidemics will come at unprecedented costs—as measured in tremendous suffering, widespread disability, and devastating financial tolls that society cannot afford.

The message I'm trying to get across here comes back full circle to the weight issue that is the focus of this book. Purely and simply, through weight control we have the power to prevent or lessen the impact of many, many cases of chronic diseases. If we as a society want to put a big dent in the incidence and severity of chronic diseases, we can successfully fight one of the biggest risk factors for many of these chronic diseases—the problem of excessive weight.

What Causes Us to Overeat?

As we try to understand what causes us to overeat, we need to look in two directions:

1. We must look inside ourselves. Some of the roots of overeating are individual issues.
2. We must look at the society in which we live—the lifestyles we live in that society, and the lifestyles of those with whom we interact.

If we want to control our weight, we must do two things:

1. We must control our own personality traits that exist deep inside ourselves that make us want to overeat and under-exercise.
2. We must "manage" our lifestyles in the society in which we live, in spite of what is going on around us. That does not mean we need to isolate ourselves from everyone. It does mean that we need to analyze what goes on around us in terms of food and eating, and make wise decisions. We don't need to, and we don't have to, go along with the trends. We need to think and plan about what we eat.

Looking Inside Ourselves about Eating

Why do people eat? People don't eat just in order to live, to stay alive. People also use food as a "tool" for some of the following reasons:

◊ Food eases depression. You might tend to overeat, or even go on eating "binges" if you're lonely, bored, or grief-stricken.

◊ Food helps relieve anxiety. You might find yourself taking in more calories if you're worried about something, if you're in the midst of making a tough decision.

◊ Food lowers barriers, lowers inhibitions. If you're a shy person, you might eat to boost your confidence to talk to others. Even if you usually aren't a shy person, you might use food to help you through a difficult time when you're making a big presentation at work, or when you're "working the crowd" at a big business or family gathering.

◊ Food is fun. In affluent societies, eating has become one of the key forums for socialization. We eat at family reunions and holiday gatherings. We go out to dinners to welcome a new staff member to our business, to congratulate a friend on an accomplishment, to get acquainted with a new neighbor, to introduce ourselves to the new "flame" in the life of our son or daughter. We eat at weddings, and we eat at funerals. The list is endless.

While all this might seem obvious, it's not really obvious. We don't give enough thought to these situations and how we will handle them on an individual basis as it relates to what we choose to eat. We have to remember that we have choices about how we handle these situations.

You don't have to overeat in order to deal with your depression. Try a little extra exercise. That will be good for you!

You don't have to overeat in order to "worry" about something. Put your energy toward solving and/or coping with the problem that's bothering you. In selected instances, put your energy toward distancing yourself from the problem if you can't solve it. Whatever you do, it's not going to help to create another problem—getting fat.

You don't have to overeat in order to lower your inhibitions. Read a good book on steps you can take to lower your inhibitions. Get some advice from a professional about this. You're not going to get more popular by getting fat.

And, finally, the fun part of eating: You can still participate in social situations that revolve around food. Just make some wise choices about what you eat, and how much you eat. Don't let others in social situations dictate what you eat.

Remember, overeating can become an addiction, just like alcohol or cigarettes. Analyze yourself and why you eat and what you eat. Then make your own wise choices.

Looking at Lifestyles of Society in Which We Live

We can't change the eating and exercise habits of the society in which we live. However, we can make our own eating and exercise habits much healthier even when we are surrounded by unhealthy lifestyles.

The first step in taking control of our own destiny is to understand some of the unhealthy eating and exercise habits to which we and our children are exposed.

If we just find our way around some of the following unhealthy habits, we can make tremendous progress in avoiding the cycle of too much eating and too little exercise:

◊ **Many adults and children have diets that include large amounts of fast foods—which mean large amounts of fatty, high-calorie foods.**

We are a fast-food society—not only in America, but in many other affluent nations as well.

The more fast food you eat, the heavier you tend to be. There's a direct correlation. One national study that extended over a 15-year period showed that the more a person increases his or her intake of fast food, the more the weight increased.

Let's just look at the United States in terms of this fast-food trend. One of the reasons Americans eat so much fast food is convenience. People are working. In a large percentage of homes, both the father and the mother are working. Folks don't want to cook the way they used to, and they are stretched to find the time and energy to cook. Thus, there's a lot of fast food.

In my years of medical practice, I ran into this situation so many times. I came to believe that the average wife and mother nowadays doesn't want a stove; instead, she wants a drive-though window.

Some results of this fast-food trend? There are increases in total calories taken in. There's an increase in intake of fat, because fast food is associated with fat. Think of it. There are few fast foods that will come to your mind that are not high in fat. Pizza, hamburgers, hot dogs....I do believe if some people really thought about this they wouldn't eat so much of this stuff. Take hot dogs, for instance. A typical single hot dog generally will yield three-quarters of a test tube of grease!!

What can you do about all this? One thing you can do is think and plan. Look around for food options that have fewer calories and less fat. They're out there—even if you're looking for something quick and convenient. Because being overweight is such a problem, some of the fast-food chains now are offering "healthier" alternatives. Check some of these out. Some are valid—meaning some really are healthier. Some are not. If you think about it, and check them out, you'll find healthier alternatives. The important thing is to think about it and look around. Don't just eat the most convenient foods regardless of the amount of calories and fat you're putting into your body (and into the bodies of your children).

◊ **There is a trend toward eating larger portions of foods—"Supersizing."**

One of the biggest eating trends today that's causing excessive weight gain is "supersizing"—over-sized portions of food.

In today's society, it's not just the foods we eat that are making us fat. It's also the huge portions of those foods.

"Supersizing" is a marketing tool that restaurants are using in order to lure customers. This is a tool being used by fast-food restaurants and by some more formal eateries as well.

Many of these supersized helpings are as much as twice as big as portions of similar foods tended to be 10 years ago. A real leader in this supersizing trend is the United States. In recent years, many visitors who have come to the U.S. from Europe have been really shocked at the size of the portions we eat. However, now some of the European restaurants are following suit. They're also serving the supersized portions.

This trend of oversized portions was among weight-related issues addressed in a federally sponsored report released in early 2006, conducted by the Keystone Center and funded by the Food and Drug Administration (FDA). This report suggested to restaurants that they look at healthier and lower-calorie menu options such as fruits and vegetables, that they provide consumers with more nutritional information about what they are eating, *and* that they consider smaller and more reasonable food portions.

But then consumers have to do their part as well. It's not only what a restaurant offers on the menu. It's also what the consumer selects. If you as a consumer allow yourself to be lured in by supersized portions, then you risk the danger of getting fat and staying fat.

For hypothetical purposes, let's just say that you have found a great restaurant that serves healthy food. You feel comfortable with the calorie count. It does not have a high fat content. The only thing is that you get these supersized portions. I have a suggestion: Split your supersized meal with a friend or family member. Or take some of it home with you, and make two meals out of it. Don't just sit there and stuff yourself with it just because the restaurant makes it available to you. Take your destiny into your own hands.

◊ **Lack of exercise is a prevalent problem.**

Just as overeating contributes to excessive weight gain, so does a lifestyle that does not have enough healthy exercise.

Lack of exercise is a huge problem, in both adults and children. And that's true in many affluent societies around the globe. Take the United Kingdom, for example. Studies have shown that in the United Kingdom over the last ten years, the average body weights have increased by about 10 percent without an increase in calories. The reason is that in the United Kingdom more people now own automobiles. As a result, many British citizens are walking less than in the past. Even in running errands near their homes, such as going to a nearby store or bank or restaurant, they are more likely to drive their automobiles instead of maybe walking a few hundred yards as they used to do. And, with the reduced exercise, they are putting on weight.

In no segment of our population is the lack of exercise a bigger problem than among our children. When I was growing up, we used to go outside and play. Nowadays, in the majority of households mothers work outside the home. And that changes the dynamics of the household, including the schedules of the children. Only a small percentage of families in this country have the traditional father/mother model of days gone by, in which the mother stayed at home. The result is that during the after-school afternoon hours many children are supervised by individuals other than their parents, and in many cases the children have no after-school adult supervision at home. Many kids come home from school and become what we call "latchkey kids"—that is, kids who are instructed by their parents to remain indoors, for safety reasons. So, instead of going outdoors and engaging in physical activity that will exercise the body and run off some calories, the kids sit indoors and play video games and computer games and/or watch television. As they watch television, the kids are inundated by advertisements for fast food and carbonated drinks that are high in calories. I mean, you're not likely to see television advertisements for carrots and lettuce or lean meat. You just don't see that.

So what are some solutions? First of all, if any of this situation applies to your children, think about it. The first step is to make yourself aware of it. Then, within the realities of your own situation—your schedule, your family budget, etc.—start planning with your children how to better manage their diet and exercise. I really do believe that if more parents would really think about this, they would find their own ways to do something about it.

Chapter 8

Confronting Your Own Moment of Truth

If you are overweight and you really want to confront your weight problem, ask yourself two questions: (1) How long do I want to live? (2) How healthy do I want to be for the rest of my life?

Obviously, even if you get your weight in line, you still will not have any "guarantees" in life. Even at a healthy weight, you can't control all your vulnerabilities as they relate to illness, disease, accident, or violence. You can't live forever. We all know that.

However, if you are overweight—and particularly if you are severely overweight, that is, obese—by losing weight you automatically shift the odds much more in your favor in terms of your health status and your longevity. To get a picture of why that's true, just refer back to Chapter 7 and to the many major health problems in which being overweight plays a factor.

I feel it appropriate here to repeat a question I posed earlier in this book: How many severely overweight older adults do you run into? Not many! (I'm referring to older adults who live into their 80s and 90s.) Severely overweight people just don't tend to live as long as thinner people.

So, if you want to be around to enjoy the fruits of what you've worked for, and if you want to spend quality time with your family (including your grandchildren, and perhaps even your great-grandchildren), ask yourself: "How long do I want to be around?" and also "How long do I want to be around with *quality?*"

By getting a handle on your weight, by getting your weight under control, you *increase* your chances of living longer with quality of life. And you *decrease* your risks of allowing too much weight and too little exercise to invalidate many of your hopes and dreams.

The Main Reasons People Lose Weight

During my 38 years as a physician, I've seen people decide to confront their weight problems mainly for the following reasons:

◊ **Concern about health**—either facing the fact they are at risk for weight-related health problems, or actually already experiencing some of these health problems.

◊ **Vanity**—concern about physical appearance, including their self-image about their weight and also concern about how others view them.

◊ **Lack of energy and lack of stamina**—frustration about not being able to "hold out" to do the things they want to do.

◊ **Desire for advancement**—including a desire to climb the ladder in the business world. There's no doubt that the workplace is not as kind to fat people in general as it is to thinner people. Overweight women in particular have a more difficult time getting hired for jobs, retaining jobs, and advancing in their work.

What Should Be Your Number One Motivator to Lose Weight?

In my mind, if you're overweight and you are mustering the get-up-and-go to confront your problem, the main motivator you *should* have is concern about your health!!

The most pressing motivator that overweight people should have to lose weight is not for aesthetics; it should not be to look better.

The most pressing motivator for weight loss should not be to feel better, to have more energy and more stamina.

Nor should the most pressing motivator for weight loss be a desire to attain some kind of advancement.

Instead, the biggest motivator for overweight people to lose weight should be, plainly and simply, to improve the status of your health. (The "bonus" is that if you lose the weight, you stand to gain in these other areas as well—satisfying your vanity, feeling better, and having a better shot at success.)

I have very strong reasons for selecting "health concern" as your most constructive weight-control motivator. First of all, potential damage to your health is *the most serious threat* you face from allowing yourself to be overweight or perhaps even obese. Also, if you are really driven to control your weight because you're concerned about your health, I believe you are more likely to live a healthy lifestyle and to be a healthier person. In fact, if you lose weight and keep it off because you are concerned about your health, I am convinced the following positive attitudes can become a part of you and your life:

◊ You will be more likely to select a *healthy and workable* diet and exercise program to get your weight off and keep it off.

◊ You are more likely to have it impressed in your mind month after month and year after year that being overweight indeed is dangerous to your health.

◊ You will be more likely to become informed about many rules of preventive medicine as they apply to you and to partner with your physician in managing your health. If you're driven to eat and exercise in a healthy manner because you care about your health, you likely won't stop there. You're likely to extend that to other areas of taking care of your health—ranging from wearing seatbelts and driving safely, to avoiding substance abuse, to getting plenty of rest, to having regular physician checkups to monitor your well-being. Getting that weight under control because you care about your health can turn out to be just a healthy first step toward a healthier you.

When "Concern" about Health Turns to FEAR

Human nature being what it is, all too many overweight people wait until they experience a crisis before they confront the health-related dangers of those extra pounds they are carrying.

They wait until they get a bad health report, or until they're having symptoms of a weight-related problem, or until they actually are diagnosed with such a problem.

In these situations, one's "concern" about weight and its health dangers can easily convert to plain old FEAR!

I know from personal experience how this fear feels. As I have detailed in this book, I didn't confront my own overweight condition until I discovered that my blood pressure was so outrageously high that I was a sitting duck to have a stroke or a heart attack at any minute!

Unfortunately, there are many of us who have to experience some kind of shock, or "kick," to really be motivated to confront being overweight and change our lifestyles.

Allow me to share some insights that might help you not to be one of those who "pushes it to the limit" before losing those extra pounds.

Not Waiting until Crisis Hits Home

Many people still fail to practice prevention when it comes to their own health—that is, preventing major health disasters they have never experienced. This goes for prevention of most any kind—taking pills to lower cholesterol, breaking the habit of smoking cigarettes, avoiding the consumption of too much alcohol. And, yes, losing weight.

Even if deep down inside individuals know they are at high risk for certain health disasters, many of them think they will somehow escape. When a person doesn't feel like he or she is sick, the attitude is likely to be, "I'm okay. Why do I need to consult with a doctor? Why do I need to stop smoking cigarettes? Why do I need to lose weight?"

I can't tell you how many times I've seen this type of attitude in patients. These are some typical scenarios:

◊ Let's say that an individual has very high cholesterol, and his physician prescribes a pill for him to take to control the condition. If this person is not experiencing symptoms, chances are pretty high that he or she won't comply in taking the cholesterol-lowering pill as instructed. However, if this same person suffers a heart attack and his physician prescribes the same cholesterol-lowering pill, chances are much better that the person will take the pill every day!

◊ Let's say another individual has several risk factors for diabetes. And this individual starts putting on weight. It's hard to convince that person to push away from the table and to spend more time exercising. And then the predicted comes: The person is diagnosed with Type 2 diabetes. Then it's much easier to do the selling job for losing weight.

I strongly urge you not to be one who has to suffer a weight-related health problem before you will do anything about your weight.

Overcoming Denial and Rationalizing

Because it's so difficult for some people to lose weight and keep it off, many overweight people wrap themselves in a cloak of denial or rationalization, or both.

People will deny to themselves that they are fat, even when they really know they are. Overeating can become an addiction, just like gambling or alcohol or cigarettes. Individuals will hang on to an overeating addiction for dear life! And they are grateful to those who help them to hold on. For example, many overweight people will "feed" off of false assurances from colleagues who fuel the denial, by making enabling comments such as "Oh, I think you look better with some weight on you," or "Goodness, you're not fat. I love you like you are."

As for rationalizing, I've seen patients come up with all kinds of excuses not to lose weight—even when the weight has reached a life-threatening level. One of the most disturbing examples that comes to my mind is a patient I met very soon after I joined the medical faculty at the School of Medicine at the University of Alabama at Birmingham (UAB).

This patient to whom I refer was a very, very obese lady. My UAB colleagues and I were very concerned about her. She was so massively obese that her life was in danger. She in fact was so obese that conventional diet and exercise were not a viable option. So I really was seriously trying to convince her to consider undergoing weight-loss surgery. Although the surgery itself was fairly dangerous, this woman's situation on the other hand was so precarious that if she did not lose weight quite soon her life expectancy was very short. However, even with knowing that her extreme weight was placing her close to death's door, this is what this lady told one of the UAB medical students who saw her: "You see, I'm so fat that I can't even walk the short distance to my mailbox and back; I have to take the car and drive 50 yards to my mailbox to get my mail, and then drive the car back. Because of my weight, I don't get much pleasure in life. The only pleasure I really get is to go out and eat. If I have this weight-loss surgery,

I have been informed that I will get physically sick if I overeat. This means that if I have the surgery and later go out to dinner and eat the kind of really big meal that I enjoy, I will proceed to get sick. As soon as I overeat, I'll start throwing up. Then I will begin to feel that I cannot comfortably go out to eat anymore. Now, if my going out to eat is taken away, I will feel that I have no pleasures left in life. So I have decided to stay as I am and just let things turn out however they may."

Making Your Own Decisions about Eating

I've seen all too many situations in which people got fat, and stayed fat, partly because of the unhealthy desires or lifestyles of other people.

Some of the most common examples are seen in people who get fat because they pick up the unhealthy eating habits of individuals with whom they interact. For example, a person might be thin and healthy and not inclined to overeat until he or she starts living with a roommate or spouse who eats too much food and also the wrong foods. So this individual who formerly had no weight problem at all finds himself or herself drawn into a lifestyle of consuming fried, fatty foods at regular meals and indulging in between-meal snacks of cookies, candies, popcorn, potato chips, and sugar-laced sodas.

Too, there are the situations in which friends or co-workers might encourage you to snack at the office and eat over-indulgent lunches. (Beware of associates who can't be happy unless *you* are eating and drinking as much as *they* are eating and drinking.)

Among the more disturbing situations I've seen are those in which people actually *want* someone to be overweight for some reason or another. For example, I've seen such circumstances occur in romantic relationships. I've seen cases in which a person proclaimed a partner to be more attractive when that partner was significantly overweight—even when that overweight condition was threatening to the partner's health. Too, I've actually met insecure men who felt more comfortable with overweight wives, because they said they didn't feel as threatened that their ladies would be stolen away from them by other men.

If you are an overweight person who is under the influence of a situation similar to one I'm describing here, I can only advise you to confront that fact and get some help to deal with your situation. Find a way to *drive your own destiny about what you eat and drink.*

Learning from Someone Else's Experience

One of the best tips I believe I can give you about confronting your overweight problem is for you to learn from someone else's weight-related healthcare crisis.

You don't have to wait to have your own crisis. You can muster up your motivation by learning from a distance what another overweight person has experienced firsthand.

My guess is that you won't have to look far to find such an experience. Many of you who are plagued with the problem of being overweight already know of a family member or friend who was decidedly overweight at the time he or she experienced a heart attack or stroke or was diagnosed with diabetes or severe joint damage.

I also invite you to learn from *my* experience. That's a key reason I wrote this book.

Taking Inventory about Yourself

If you are concerned about being overweight, it can be very enlightening for you to take inventory of what's going on with your body.

This means that you should confront how big you are. It also means that you should take some simple health-screening tests that will tell you how your body is functioning.

Confronting Your Size

This can be tough. I know that I personally found it very difficult to summon the courage to step on the scales soon after I confronted the reality that I had to lose weight. However, if you are going to confront your own weight problem, you must form a bond with the scales. You can't really deal with your weight problem until you know the *extent* of your weight problem.

If you have not already done so, you need to weigh yourself on some accurate, reliable scales. And if you have not already done so, you need to measure yourself around the middle.

Weighing yourself regularly and often is all-important at every stage of the weight-management process. Stepping on the scales is important when you're first confronting your weight problem. It's important when you're in the midst of a weight-loss program. It's important after you reach your targeted weight and are focused on maintaining that weight. It's just plain important. You must know where you are with your weight. As for how much you should weigh according to your height and body frame, you can find some guidelines in Chapter 2, under the subheading of "How Much Should I Weigh?" You also can find guidelines in a chart in the back of the book.

Measuring yourself is also crucial. Get out the tape measure and measure your waist. Make sure that you measure your waistline honestly, by placing the tape measure at the correct place on your body. Place the tape measure at the level of your umbilicus (navel). Resist the temptation to place the tape measure considerably up or down from your navel. Placing the tape measure well below the navel could be especially tempting to many men (especially overweight men) who might wear their pants a considerable distance below their navel. If these men measure where they wear their pants, they likely will get a much smaller waist size than by measuring at navel level. How much is *too much* to be showing on that measurement of the waistline? If the waist of a woman measures more than 35 inches, or if the waist of a man measures more than 40 inches, that can be an indication this person is at high risk to already be suffering from a condition that we refer to as "metabolic syndrome" or "insulin-resistance syndrome." Individuals who have this condition have as much as five times the rate of heart disease.

Checking Out the "Numbers"

In addition to finding out how much you weigh and how much your waistline measures, you need to visit your physician to undergo three simple health-screening tests that will reveal the "numbers" about what's going on inside your body.

These are the three tests:

- ◊ Get your blood pressure checked.
- ◊ Get your blood sugar checked.
- ◊ Get your cholesterol checked.

Just getting the results of these three health-screening tests—plus knowing your weight and your waistline measurement—might well be enough for a complete "confrontation" where your weight is concerned. This inventory might be enough for you to tell yourself, "Wow! I'm really not invulnerable." It might be enough for you to sit down with your physician and start planning the weight-loss program that can work best for you.

Chapter 9

Embarking On Your Own Weight-Loss Program

If you are overweight and you have made the decision to shed some pounds, I strongly advise you *to search out and select a weight-loss program that is tailored just for your own needs.* Diets and exercise programs are not generic. The same diet won't fit every person. The same exercise program won't fit every person.

Don't play "follow the leader" and blindly adopt someone else's weight-loss plan. That advice applies to my own weight-loss plan that I described in Chapter 2 of this book as well as anyone else's plan. While I believe my One-Plus-One Weight-Loss Plan will work for many people, I also believe it will not match the needs of many others.

When I decided to write this book, my goals were (1) to motivate many overweight people to lose weight, and (2) to arm them with information on *how* to lose weight. My description of my own One-Plus-One Weight-Loss Plan is only *part* of that information.

While I hope there will be readers of this book who will use and benefit from my One-Plus-One Plan, I also hope there will be many readers who choose other weight-loss plans who also will find helpful weight-loss information in this book.

Selecting a Diet You Can Follow for a Lifetime

When you are selecting a weight-loss program, remember that it should be a long-term guide, not a short-term guide.

Your weight-loss program should, in fact, be a program you can live with for the rest of your life—to lose the weight, and then to keep the weight off, in a healthy manner. In selecting a weight-loss plan that is tailored for your needs, the number one thing that you must ask yourself is, "Can I live with this program over the long-term?"

In Chapter 2 of this book, I explained that when I was devising my own weight-loss plan in 2003, I sort of viewed it as a long-term deal much in the way one should think when choosing a spouse.

What we're talking about here is not some temporary, short-term weight-loss plan to help you fit into a tuxedo or a dress for a wedding. We're not talking about some quick-fix plan you use during the month of January to get off the weight you gained during Christmas.

Where the diet portion of your plan is concerned, your best shot is a diet that will lower your calorie intake while at the same time give you a healthy, balanced intake of food—food choices heavy with fresh fruits and vegetables, mingled with poultry and fish if you like, very little bread, and virtually no desserts (preferably *no* desserts).

And, remember that your weight-loss plan must have not just one part, but two parts. The plan should not just be dieting. It also should be regular, healthy, and effective exercise.

"Quick Fixes" and "Helpmates" to Promote Weight Loss

If losing weight and keeping weight off were easy, then there wouldn't be so many fat people and there would be no need for a book like this. I've said it before, and I'll say it again: *Losing weight and keeping it off is not for wimps!*

All too many people suffer negative results when they reach out for the "quick fix" to lose weight. Some of them end up gaining weight rather than losing. Others might drop a lot of weight and then quickly gain it back. And there are those who actually damage their health in some way with one of these quick fixes. Remember those days when patients were rushing out to get amphetamine-like weight-loss pills, and as a result some of them suffered dangerous, sometimes deadly, heart-related problems?

Let's take a look at some of these alleged quick fixes and helpmates:

Fad Diets

I really am opposed to these fad diets in which you eat only certain foods or you go out and buy some kind of powdered concoction. So someone tells you that you can lose weight if you eat only strawberries and skim milk for six weeks, or only bananas? Or you hear about some highly promoted "nutritional supplement" that you're supposed to stay on for several weeks or months. So how are you going to have a healthy diet that you can stay on for a lifetime if you're out there eating mainly strawberries or bananas or all these powdered mixtures? What's going to happen after you drop a few pounds and then you return to your "normal" eating? I'll tell you what. You're very likely going to regain the weight.

I also place the "fad diet" label on very unbalanced diets that are unhealthy. These are diets in which one goes to the extreme to totally eliminate a class of foods from the diet that should not be eliminated. These are weight-loss programs in which foods are eliminated from the diet to the extent the body is deprived of some of the essential vitamins, minerals, and other nourishment it needs. As a physician, I'll tell you that high on my list of complaints here is any diet that totally eliminates carbohydrates. We need a small amount of carbohydrates in our diet. My vote is for a low-carbohydrate diet, not a no-carbohydrate diet. In explaining why I included a small amount of carbohydrates in my own diet, I discussed the potential side effects of no-carbohydrates in Chapter 2 of this book, in a section entitled "A Word About Carbohydrates and Me." To refresh your memory, some of the potential side effects of no-carbohydrate diets include a rise in cholesterol levels, disruption in normal metabolism, hair loss, a very unpleasant fruity-smelling breath, a sluggish feeling, severe constipation, and heart arrhythmias.

Gastric bypass surgery

Gastric bypass surgery is an extreme choice that's out there to fit extreme situations. It's an option that should be considered only in a case of very severe obesity, and only when the person is facing major health risks associated with obesity. Gastric bypass surgery certainly is not for routine weight loss. Before you take the gastric bypass surgery option, make sure you have excellent medical advice, avail yourself of more than one medical opinion, select a top-notch surgeon, and retain the services of a well-qualified physician who knows your own health issues well and who can follow you medically both before and after you undergo gastric bypass surgery.

Non-Prescription Weight-Loss Products

In regard to products advertised to help you lose weight, I strongly advise you to beware of what I refer to as the "snake-oil salesmen" and their "miracle weight-loss" advertisements. These are the salespeople who are likely to show up on late-night and weekend television ads, and in-print advertisements as well, and who tout this or that product as your easy path to losing lots of weight quickly. These are products you can obtain without a physician's prescription. They range from pills to sprays, creams, liquid extracts, patches, what have you. Some are touted as being some kind of miracle herbal supplement, as being a product of some rare tree or shrub, or a secret recipe from some exotic island or "research lab." In peddling these products, the manufacturers claim they can do everything from reducing your appetite and reining in your food cravings to controlling your blood sugar, speeding up your metabolism, and giving you more energy. Some of these products are sold through mail-order, via print advertisements, or through TV or internet marketing. Others can be purchased in conventional consumer outlets; you simply go into a store and buy them. *Beware of these bogus products. Not only do you stand to throw your money away on useless products; you also could damage your health with some of this garbage!* I will tell you plainly and simply that I agree strongly with this warning about such products that has been published by the U.S. Food and Drug Administration (FDA): "Products and programs that promise quick and easy weight loss are bogus. To lose weight, you have to lower your intake of calories and increase your physical activity." I agree with a similar warning that comes from the Federal Trade Commission. "Flip through a magazine, scan a newspaper, or channel surf and you see them everywhere. Ads that promise quick and easy weight loss without diet or exercise. Wouldn't it be nice if—as the ads claim—you could lose weight simply by taking a pill, wearing a patch, or rubbing in a cream? Too bad claims like that are almost always false." (In underscoring warnings from the FDA and Federal Trade Commission, overall I would advise you to evaluate these weight-loss "miracle" products with this often-quoted adage in mind: "If it sounds too good to be true, usually it is *not* true.")

Every once in a while you will run across an over-the-counter aid for weight-loss that might have some limited benefit. But most of the time you will also have to deal with some side effects as well. One example is a class of over-the-counter medications that block the breakdown of fat in the gut. You'd better check these out carefully and think about them before you take them. On the one hand, these medications cut down on absorption of calories because fat passes straight through the gastric intestinal tract and is not broken down the way it usually is. On the other hand, some people taking this type of medication have experienced very unpleasant "accidents"—suddenly passing greasy diarrhea-like fluid.

Prescription Weight-Loss Products

There are some legitimate prescription medications that can help some selected patients in a weight-loss program. Additional prescription medications are being investigated for possible future approval and distribution. However, these medications are not for all persons. Some of them, in fact, are designed only for individuals who have specific diseases, such as diabetes. In my own weight-loss program, I used no weight-loss products at all, including no prescription medications related to weight loss. I believe the majority of patients who go on a weight-loss program should not and would not be candidates for weight-loss medications. Even if a person is a candidate for one of these prescription medications, the medication alone won't weave the weight-loss magic. In addition to the medication, the person still will need to maintain a good diet-and-exercise program. Too, before taking any of these prescription medications, the consumer should proceed very carefully and make sure he or she really is a candidate for such a medication. We all know that just because a medication can be obtained through a physician's prescription, this does not mean that a given medication is safe or appropriate for every individual. Before taking a prescription medication, check it out carefully and work closely with a top-flight physician.

When I think of already approved prescription medications on the market that can be a tool to help some individuals with weight-loss, two that come to my mind, specifically for persons with Type 2 diabetes, are Metformin® and Byetta®. Both work to control blood sugar levels and in the process can help with weight control. Again, neither is for every individual who has Type 2 diabetes.

In another group of weight-related prescription drugs, there are some modern-day versions of the amphetamine-like appetite suppressants; I call them "speed" derivatives. While some of these modern-day appetite suppressants might be safer than the dangerous amphetamine drugs of yesteryear, I still feel that they have very temporary action in suppressing appetite. After you've taken them for three to six months, I don't think you'll get much benefit from them.

Working with Your Physician

To anyone undertaking a major weight-loss program, I would advise strongly that you work closely with a qualified physician who knows your medical history and who can monitor you medically during your weight-loss program. This is especially important if you have health conditions that need to be monitored, and/or if you are planning to lose a substantial amount of weight.

Keep in mind you could have health conditions you don't even know about that would need to be managed in conjunction with your weight-loss program. You could have diabetes, high blood pressure, heart problems, any number of situations that could get you into trouble if you just go marching out there on a major weight-loss program with no medical monitoring.

When I was losing weight, I worked with a physician I consider qualified and one who certainly knew my medical history well. I emerged from my weight-loss program in good shape, and as far as I can tell I continue to be in good health. However, I probably should have consulted a different physician other than the one I chose. The reason is that the physician I used was myself! I've heard it said that only a fool uses himself as his own physician. I will tell you that in recent months I have engaged a physician other than myself.

So why do you need a physician to monitor you in conjunction with a weight-loss program? There are several things a physician can do for you:

◊ **Health screenings.** Your physician can coordinate your obtaining those all-important up-front screenings, such as checking your cholesterol, your blood sugar, and your blood pressure. These screenings need to be conducted *before* you start a weight-loss program.

◊ **Motivation.** Your physician can explain to you the health reasons for you to lose weight—that is, give you that little bit of extra motivation.

◊ **Diet and exercise consultation.** Your physician can work with you to find the diet and exercise program that suits you best. Now, you might come in with some suggestions. However, you can get valuable medical input from your physician as to whether a given diet plan or exercise plan is the right one medically for *You*!

◊ **Managing your health conditions.** While you're dieting and exercising, you need the medical supervision of your physician to closely monitor and manage any health problems you have. Embarking on a diet and exercise program will not take the place of medications and other treatment you need for conditions such as diabetes, high blood pressure, and heart problems. Also, when you begin losing weight, your body can undergo changes in relation to certain health conditions and the dosages of your medicines might need to be adjusted accordingly.

Take diabetes, for example. When you have diabetes and you start to lose weight, your body tends to become more sensitive to insulin. If you are on therapies to lower your blood sugar, you can in effect get quite low blood sugars after you start dieting and exercising and losing weight. If you are a person with diabetes who is in the process of losing weight, you must have a physician who can monitor the dosages of your diabetes medications to see if those dosages need to be altered.

Blood pressure is another medical situation that can undergo changes as you lose weight. With substantial weight loss, blood pressure can drop quite significantly. When you are dieting, you might find that you will suddenly get dizzy when you stand up from a chair or when you first get out of bed in the morning, because your blood pressure is too low. Therefore, if you are taking blood pressure control medicines they might need to be adjusted.

◊ **Monitoring your weight loss and how your body reacts.** From an exercise view, your physician will want to keep tabs on whether you're putting too much stress on your heart, your joints, etc. From a diet view, if you're dropping a lot of pounds, your physician likely will want to keep close tabs on some of your bodily chemistries. In conjunction with your weight-loss program, you might need some supplements here and there. These are some examples of what might be monitored chemistry-wise:

1. What we call a "renal profile"—sodium, potassium, etc.

2. Your blood count. A close look needs to be taken here at iron levels in the blood. There are some people who don't take in enough iron when they go on a diet, so they need iron supplementation. You know, we really don't have access to a wide variety of good food sources of iron, other than meat and liver and that kind of thing. In general, women run a greater risk than men to develop a low iron level when they are dieting, because women have such low iron stores to start with. A situation of too-little iron is very easily corrected. With some of my own patients who have become iron-deficient, I have at times used intravenous iron to bolster their iron stores.

3. Measuring vitamin D levels. While I would hope that dieters would select diets that provide a lot of calcium and vitamin D intake, you want to make sure you're getting enough calcium and vitamin D. Since we know that some dieters do sustain a decrease in vitamin D, your doctor would want to measure your vitamin D levels—to ensure that problems which could cause bone diseases do not develop.

4. Some extra monitoring for the gastric bypass surgery patient. In the cases of people who undergo gastric bypass surgery, we find that we need to carefully monitor their blood count (including looking at iron levels), their vitamin D levels, and also their B-12 and folic acid levels.

Battling More than One Addiction at Once

I'm all for self-improvement. But then, I'm also all for being realistic.

During my years as a physician, I've seen people become over-zealous about tackling too many self-improvement projects at once. If you put too much on yourself, you can well set yourself up for failure on all fronts.

Along these lines, I have a piece of advice for you: If you are undertaking a major weight-loss program, do not tackle more than one addiction at once. In particular that means don't try to lose weight and stop smoking at the same time.

Overeating and smoking cigarettes are both addictions. You might get in the frame of mind to make some positive changes in your life and decide, "Well, I'm going to put down these cigarettes, and at the same time I'm going to embark on a weight-loss plan to lose 75 pounds!"

This is what you should do: Make a choice about which addictive-habit you want to deal with first. Once you've kicked one addiction, give yourself six months to a year and then say, "Now is the time to handle the other one."

I'll tell you this positive aspect: Kicking one habit will likely give you a boost toward being successful at kicking the second habit. If you lose weight or you quit smoking, that can magnify your confidence to go ahead and get rid of the second problem.

As an aside, I'm convinced that cigarette smoking is an addiction much more difficult to deal with than overeating. In fact, cigarette smoking is such a strong, terrible addiction that I believe for some individuals cigarette smoking is an addiction more difficult to break than alcohol or even street drugs. A friend of mine who was a heavy smoker once told me, "David, if I could just get past 10 o'clock in the morning, I just know I could give up cigarettes. But I can never get past 10 o'clock in the morning without lighting up a cigarette." Well, the first morning he got beyond 10 o'clock without a cigarette was the morning he suffered a heart attack and was rushed to the hospital. That also was the day he quit smoking.

As I've told you previously in this book, I smoked cigarettes for a few years before giving them up in my late 20s when my father, a smoker, was diagnosed with terminal lung cancer. Years later I picked up a pipe-smoking habit. About 16 years ago, when I was in my mid-40s, I laid down my pipe for good after I suffered chest pains and feared I had heart problems. (My health problem at the time turned out to be an inflamed esophagus.) I bring this up to note that I can identify somewhat with smokers. However, fortunately I was not addicted in a major way to cigarette smoking and was able to give up cigarettes; and later I had no trouble stopping the pipe-smoking.

If you are a *fat smoker*, you are really at risk for a lot of health problems. Being fat puts you at risk. Smoking puts you at risk. Put them together and you are aiming two potentially lethal weapons at yourself. You don't need to smoke. You don't need to be fat. At the same time, in order to break both habits you're going to have to put forth a little more self-discipline than the average person. In deciding which habit you want to tackle first, this is a reality you must keep in mind: There is no doubt that many smokers tend to gain weight after they stop smoking. If you already are fat before you stop smoking, once you stop smoking you likely will have to work even harder to bring that weight under control and keep it there. My own personal experience along these lines was that after I quit my pipe-smoking habit, I proceeded to put on a good deal of weight! The tobacco habit that is so bad for you on the one hand actually has some up-sides on the weight-control side. Smoking increases your metabolism, so you burn up more calories. Also, when you smoke, you tend to eat less because (1) you can't taste food as keenly as a non-smoker, and (2) you are likely to want to hurry up and finish eating so you can smoke.

It actually has been said that some smokers—particularly women—make a conscious decision to continue smoking because they fear they will gain weight if they quit. Bad decision!

Tips about Your Dieting

In order to have a healthy, effective diet that you can use to lose weight and keep it off, start out by thinking in four categories:

1. Building on your favorite foods.
2. Controlling your portions.
3. Striking a healthy balance.
4. Breaking bad eating habits.

These are a few tips:

Building on Your Top 20 Foods

You'll have a good start toward a healthy, effective diet you can live with the rest of your life if you come up with a diet that (1) you like, and that (2) has some familiarity.

Many of you can find that appeal and familiarity in foods that you already have been eating.

The truth of the matter is that the majority of people already have a regular diet that is headed up by the same 20 foods they have eaten regularly for much of their lives. For many of you, if you just think about it logically and sit down and make a list, you will not get beyond 20 foods that you eat regularly or even frequently. (And in most cases I believe the majority of your top 20 foods will be common ones. I mean, how many of you will have lobster thermidor on your list? I know that I did not have it on *my* list!)

The chances are that as you structure your new diet to lose weight, you will be able to retain at least a few, and perhaps *quite* a few, of these 20 foods that are familiar and appealing to you.

Actually, your goal should be to retain in your new diet as many as possible of the foods that are both familiar and appealing to you. It just stands to reason that the more changes you have to make in your daily menu, the more will-power you will have to exert. If you change someone's diet toward something that is altogether unfamiliar, within a few weeks the body is going to want to go back to the previous diet.

So, list your top 20 foods and start the process:

◊ Eliminate foods that clearly are not beneficial. The first foods that will have to go will be heavy desserts! Then take a sharp pen to energy-dense carbohydrates. Do not eliminate carbohydrates entirely. Just use your wisdom. You know some things that need to be cut. Remember that when you drop a calorie-dense carbohydrate such as bread or potatoes you can compensate with a fruit or vegetable. (When I made my own list, I knew the first thing that had to go—too much bread!) You might find that you'll end up eating the same amount of protein you've been accustomed to eating, and perhaps close to the same amount of fruits and vegetables that you have been eating.

◊ If you eat frequently in restaurants—and particularly if you are a regular customer of fast-food restaurants—you're going to have to make some strong choices there. For example, those high-fat, high-calorie hamburgers and French fries will have to go! On the positive side, increasing numbers of restaurants (including fast-food restaurants) are now offering menu options with fewer calories, less fat, and smaller portions. Search out those options and avail yourself of them!

Controlling Your Portions

After you decide which foods you need to eat as part of your weight-control program, you must zero in on limiting the amounts of these foods that you consume.

There is no way to emphasize enough the need to cut back on portions. In civilized, affluent societies, we simply tend to eat portions of food that are way too large if our goal is to keep our weight under control.

At the family dinner table, forget about going back for all those second and third helpings. When you eat in restaurants, you must start evaluating the portions that are served to you. If the restaurant portions are too big, don't eat all that food; take some of it home and make two meals out of it. Take home a "doggie bag," even if you don't have a dog!

Striking a Healthy Balance

Since I made my own life-changing decision to lose weight, these are some of the guides I have used to strike a healthy balance with my own eating:

◊ **Making sure to get adequate nutrition.** This means eating balanced meals that feature salads, fruits, vegetables, lean meat, poultry, and fish.

◊ **Identifying foods that will limit calorie intake and at the same time provide nutrition.** Beware of consuming a lot of foods in your diet that fail to provide you with any nutritional value. A good example here has to do with salad ingredients. In selecting the basic ingredients for a salad, you need to go for the spinach instead of the lettuce. Iceberg lettuce is nutritionally useless. Spinach is much better than any of the lettuces we use in salads.

◊ **Selecting snacks that are nutritious and not fatty.** Some of the fruits make great snacks. Apples are a great snack. Nuts that are not really salty also can be good snacks. Celery or carrots are good. I often use tomatoes as a snack. That really works for me when I'm attending a social or business event in which there is a big buffet table with fattening foods. On most any of these tables you also can find tomatoes. While a lot of other folks are wandering around the room munching on breadsticks, chips and dip, and/or several miniature desserts, I make my "talking rounds" while munching on a plate of tomatoes. The key is to zero in on snack foods that are low in calories and also tend to be filling. These foods often are called "high-satiety" foods because they have the ability to satisfy or satiate your appetite without piling on the calories.

◊ **Not just reaching for something because it's convenient.** A good example of that is a muffin. How many times do we see muffins for sale on the counter of some store? Most muffins are not what dieters should be eating. Usually they are chunked full of calories and fat, and usually sugar as well.

◊ **Finding out about foods that seem to be great for dieters, but which in reality are not!** Along these lines, a lot of people don't realize that there are three popular fruits that are the "forbidden fruits" because they are very high in carbohydrate and high in sugar content. These three fruits are bananas, pineapples, and strawberries. Now, I'm not saying don't ever eat those fruits. However, you need to realize they are not a dieter's dream.

◊ **Recognizing the downfall ingredient in many soups that appear to be healthy. That ingredient is salt.** It's very difficult to stay away from excess salt when you eat soup. At first glance, a zesty vegetable soup might look like a healthy food choice, but the downside is that most vegetable soups are all too salty. Especially when you have high-blood-pressure problems, you want to keep your salt intake to a minimum.

◊ **Limiting the intake of eggs.** You can eat eggs while you're dieting. But I suggest you limit your egg consumptions to no more than two occasions weekly.

◊ **Staying away from most bread.** I love bread. I could sit down at one meal and consume two loaves of bread. However, I have learned to severely limit my intake of bread. I advise you to do the same thing. Bread is clearly another calorie source that you can avoid.

◊ **Finding some substitutes for desserts**. If you are serious about losing weight and keeping it off, you really need to back away from desserts. I suggest you give them up entirely until you get down to your ideal weight, and then if you want an occasional dessert just make sure it's occasional. There was a time when I really overindulged on desserts. Sometimes at a single meal I would have two helpings of dessert and then finish up somebody else's dessert if he or she didn't want it! Since I embarked on my weight-control program, I have used fruit or cheese as a substitute for desserts. Actually, I've come to enjoy these dessert substitutes, and I'm not drawn to those heavy desserts like I once was. (I wish I could say I'm not still drawn to bread!!! I will forever have to fight that. In days gone by, I think bread was *my* true dessert.)

Developing Some New Eating Habits

When I speak of developing some new eating habits, I'm referring to habits that will reduce your tendency to eat too much.

These are four habits I suggest you cultivate:

◊ **Using the 20-minute rule to avoid overeating.** Did you know that it takes 20 minutes after you eat for your brain to realize that your stomach is full? If you just keep shoveling in food, with no pause, then you can be bloated with hundreds of extra calories that make you uncomfortable on the short-term and fat on the long-term. My advice to you is that when you are consuming a meal, and you have eaten what your instincts and good sense and calorie counting all tell you is sufficient, don't reach for another bite of food until 20 minutes have gone by. That's particularly a good tip for you dessert-lovers. Eat your main course. Before you decide on dessert, wait 20 minutes. By that time, you might well realize you'll full and you don't even want that dessert.

◊ **Using dental care to fight off night snacking.** I hear people talk a lot about being caught up in the habit of "night-snacking." Simply stated, this habit consists of eating snacks in the hours just before bedtime, and in some cases even getting up in the middle of the night and snacking. Of course, there is no doubt that this habit can just stack the pounds on you. I have a suggestion for you that has to do with your making it inconvenient to yourself to do that. The suggestion relates to dental care. When the evening arrives and as soon as possible after you have consumed any evening meal, conduct a thorough dental-care session. Get out your toothbrush and toothpaste and dental floss and thoroughly cleanse your teeth and gums. View that dental-care routine as your own message to yourself: You're going to keep your teeth and gums clean, and in order to do that your eating is finished for the day. This means no night-snacking in the evening while visiting with family and friends, no sitting around eating snacks while reading or watching television, no food whatsoever after you complete the last scheduled meal of the day. Establishing this routine can be great for your dental care, and it can also be great for your dieting.

◊ **Avoiding distractions that contribute to overeating.** Don't eat while you're doing something else—such as working or watching television or a movie. It has been shown clearly that, when people have these distractions, as a general rule they tend to eat more than when they do not have these distractions. If you're sitting at your desk talking on the phone or working on the computer while eating lunch, it can be very easy to cram your mouth full of everything in sight—a sandwich, potato chips, cookies, sugar-laden soft drink, whatever. On the other hand, if you're really serious about your weight-control diet and you take time out to sit down and eat a meal without distractions, you'll tend to enjoy your food more but at the same time eat less. As for watching television or a movie, just enjoy those pleasures without accompanying them with food. When you are at home watching TV, stay away from your refrigerator. When you go to the movie, take the concession stand off your list of stops.

◊ **Using your lunch hour for an exercise break instead of eating a big lunch.** In other words, this is substituting exercise for food. Now, the idea of taking a break from work in mid-day is a healthy one—to give the brain and body a rest. However, *there is nothing written down that says you have to use your lunch break to eat.* My suggestion is instead of eating during your lunch hour, you put on some walking shoes and use that hour to exercise. Once you're accustomed to this routine, many of you will find that the exercise at lunch can give you as much pleasure as eating—just in different ways. How is that true? For one thing, when you exercise you release pleasurable chemicals called endorphins, and those endorphins can lift your spirits and increase your energy level. Exercise also with most people will suppress appetite. Too, exercising during your lunch hour can bring great dividends as a time-saver. This is how the time-saving can work for you when you're involved in a serious diet and exercise program: If you're exercising daily, this of course means you must set aside a chunk of time each day for your exercise. By doing your daily exercise during the lunch hour, you accomplish two things. (1)You avoid taking in what could be hundreds of calories at lunch. (2) You free up other time periods during the day and evening that you might otherwise set aside for exercising. By doing your exercise during lunch, you don't have to get up real early in the morning to exercise. Too, since you're not designating evening hours for exercise, after you finish your daily routine you can devote your evening hours to relaxation and spending time with your family.

Tips About Your Exercise Program

It's essential that you have an exercise component to your weight-loss program if you're going to have a well-rounded, effective program. Dieting alone won't do it.

In Chapter 2 of this book, in which I outlined my own One-Plus-One Weight-Loss Plan, I explained that my two-part program consists of (1) eating one meal a day and (2) engaging in one hour of exercise a day. I also detailed the exercise regimen that I selected—a combination of walking, treadmill, and lifting weights. It just so happens that I like walking, I also like the treadmill. Although I had to become accustomed to using the weights, I'll have to say that the weights and I have become friends. I found that I needed the weights for toning my upper body, and I've been pleased with the results of using them.

As for what kind of exercise program you choose, that's up to you. As is true with your diet program, you need to come up with an exercise program that matches your tastes and lifestyle, that is healthy and matches your own health issues, that will work and produce good results, and that you can live with on the long-term. *Especially if you have health issues regarding exercise, consult with your physician before you select which type of exercise is best for you.*

I recommend that you try to have an exercise program that includes an hour of exercise a day. In terms of consistency and stickability, confront the fact that you must make a commitment to exercise. You don't need an exercise program that you fit in only when it's convenient to you. This means that you don't need to exercise only every now and then, depending on your schedule or your mood that day. Place a high priority on your exercise program. View your daily appointment with exercise with the same degree of importance that you view keeping an important professional or business appointment.

These are a few of my opinions about various types of exercise:

◊ **Exercise equipment.** I like the treadmill, and it gives you a good workout—burning up calories, good for the cardiovascular system, and strengthening your muscles, particularly in the lower body. While the treadmill exercise strengthens the muscles of your legs, it falls short in strengthening the muscles of your upper body. That's why I added weights to my exercise regimen.

Now, there are some people who have knee problems who might like a cross-country walking machine better than a treadmill. There's no question but that the cross-country walking machine is easier on the knees than the treadmill.

Then there are those who might prefer a stationary bicycle. My feeling about a stationary bicycle is that, for the effort you put out, you really can't burn up as many calories as with the treadmill. With a stationary bicycle, there's a limit to how much action you can get. You rather quickly will reach a limit as to the stress you can place on your quadriceps muscle (that large muscle in front of the thigh).

◊ **Running.** I personally am not fond of running as an exercise. There are too many injuries associated with running.

◊ **Jogging.** I have a little bit better opinion of jogging than I do of running, although not much better. I still prefer brisk walking to jogging. If you want to jog, I'd advise that you jog for a shorter time than if you were walking—maybe no more than 20 to 30 minutes per jogging session.

Too, I tend to think that generally speaking jogging should be left to the younger set. I'm not for middle-aged and senior citizens out there jogging; over-exertion and/or injury can become a problem.

◊ **Aerobics.** Aerobics is fine, if you find a good program that works for you. Some people thrive on the programmed nature of an aerobics regimen.

◊ **Water aerobics.** Water aerobics is a great exercise selection for some individuals who have health problems that prevent them from doing other types of exercise. For example, individuals who have severe arthritis can be really good candidates for water aerobics.

◊ **Walking.** In my view, I saved the best for last. I think brisk walking is the best exercise you can do. Just get out there and walk! If you walk briskly on a regular basis, that is the world's best exercise. You're not going to damage your knees; you're not going to damage your feet; you're not going to damage your back, no matter how heavy you are. Even with people who have a little arthritis in their knees, a little walking can actually help.

A few tips about your walking:

◊ **Walk within your limits.** Don't over-extend yourself.

◊ **If you're walking with a friend, a clue to being within your limits is whether or not you can carry on a conversation without exerting a lot of effort.** If you're out walking with a friend and you're too short of breath to carry on a conversation and gossip, then you're going at it too hard. That's your clue that you're over-doing it. Walk slower. Cut your walk short if you need to.

◊ **When you walk, do not use weights.** Don't carry weights, and definitely do not strap weights to your body. Especially do not strap weights to your lower legs! Those weights can lead to injury—including injuries to the joints. I don't believe the carrying-weights-while-walking exercise approach is a wise plan at all. I do not use weights while walking, and I don't recommend that others use them.

Guides to How Much You Should Weigh

Once you start losing weight, you might encounter lots of folks who will venture an opinion about your weight. You might have friends and relatives who tell you that you've lost enough, that you should eat more, and that you looked better when you were fat.

Where do you go to get valid information about how much you should weigh? Well, that's not difficult to answer. There are weight-height-body build charts out there that can give you a good guide. If you go to Chapter 2 and to a chart in the back of this book, you can get a good idea by re-reading the section in that chapter entitled "How Much Should I Weigh?" To save you from turning the pages, here's an excerpt from that section:

"If an adult male wants to figure his 'ideal weight,' this is the formula he uses: Start with a baseline of five feet in height and a weight of 106 pounds. Then, for every inch, add six pounds. That means a man who is 5 feet, 10 inches tall should weigh roughly 166 pounds.

"For a woman to calculate her 'ideal weight,' she starts with 100 pounds and five feet in height, and she adds five pounds for each inch. This means that a woman of 5 feet, 4 inches would have an "ideal weight" of 120.

"Now, this 'ideal' can vary as much as 10 percent up or down—depending on how large or small a body frame you have, and frankly, depending on how you look and feel at a given weight."

Your physician also is a good one to consult about how much you should weigh. He or she might have health-related reasons for wanting you to be a few pounds over or under the average.

When it gets beyond paying attention to the "weight-height-body build charts" and to seeking the advice of your physician, I also have a few suggestions to you about listening to other self-appointed guides about your weight:

◊ Don't be so arrogant that you totally ignore the comments of someone whose opinion you really trust. That's a real important key: Make sure a comment is coming to you for the right reasons from someone whose opinion you trust. If someone you really trust tells you that you are getting a little gaunt and perhaps have lost too much weight, seriously evaluate whether you might have taken things too far with your weight loss. Look at those weight charts. If your actual weight is in line with the charts, consider addressing any gaunt look you might have through exercise—toning up targeted body areas.

Now, my own One-Plus-One Weight-Loss Plan was so effective that I will admit that at one point I had lost a few pounds more than I needed to. Some people in my life whom I trusted told me I was a bit too thin and a little gaunt. I listened to them. In fact, their comments matched what I was seeing in the mirror. So I took two steps to adjust: First of all, I gained back 10 pounds, so that my weight matched the ideal on the charts. At the same time, I added some weight-lifting to my exercise routine to tone up and build up my upper body.

◊ Don't be so gullible that you fall victim to comments people make to you about your weight for the wrong reasons. What are some of the wrong reasons? Well, some people will tell you that you have lost too much weight because they feel uncomfortable around you because they are overweight themselves. Many overweight people would like for us to float around in the same ill-directioned boat with them. You know, I have mentioned before that I really love my patients. At the same time, I believe that over the years some of my patients have felt more comfortable with me when they saw me having the same bad habits that they had. Back when I smoked a pipe, there were times my patients would see me with the pipe in my office (before the days when the UAB Medical Center became a non-smoking environment). Well, after I quit the pipe-smoking habit I had a number of patients say, "Doc, I miss your pipe. I liked the smell of that pipe tobacco." Then, years later, when I started losing weight, I had quite a number of patients say, "Doc, don't lose any more. You're getting too thin." The truth is that for health reasons I didn't need to be smoking that pipe. And the truth is that before I made the decision to shed weight I was putting my health in severe jeopardy by being more than 100 pounds overweight. Long before I reached a healthy weight level that matched the chart's ideal for my height and body build, I was being told by some of my overweight patients that I had lost too much weight and was too thin!

◊ Recognize the trends in society that have to do with eating, and know that in order to be at a healthy weight you must muster the courage to go against some of these trends. People often will try to push you to overeat (and thus to be overweight) because of a number of trends in our society that have to do with food. Don't fall victim to these trends:

◊ Such a high percentage of people in our society today are overweight that many people have lost track of what a "normal" and "healthy" weight is!

◊ Eating too much and eating the wrong things are such a part of our socializing that often people will encourage you to eat, and eat, and eat, in order to be sociable. One example: A hostess wants you to eat lots of her food to make her feel good because she cooked the food and it's her way of showing hospitality. You need to find ways to work around that. Another example: You have friends with whom you're dining. Those friends want to try various items on the menu, including rich desserts; and they want you to join in the "feast." Again, you have to find ways to work around that.

Can you be too thin? Of course you can! But use those weight-height-body build charts, and your physician, as your guides. You'll probably have friends, family, and colleagues accuse you of being too thin long before you get there!

Get Ready, Get Set, Go!

So … did I hear you say you've made the commitment to get started with a weight-loss program?

If you're really serious, here's your "get-started kit."

◊ Have whatever consultation you need with your physician.

◊ Settle on the diet and exercise program you're going to use. Give your plan a good chance. If the program is not suiting you, and is too difficult for you, then consider another program. Remember: You need to find a program you can use for life—to get that weight off, and then to keep it off.

◊ Commit yourself to a starting date for your weight-loss program, and stick to the date you set. Don't keep putting it off by saying, "Well, I'll do it next week." Instead, say, "I'm going to start Day One (with a date attached)." Mark Day One on your calendar, and launch your program that day.

◊ Between the time you make your decision and the time you launch your weight-loss program, be careful not to "over-celebrate." In other words, don't stuff yourself with food and gain even more weight before you start the weight-loss program. You don't need the extra pounds. Too, before you start dieting, you don't need to get accustomed to even more overeating.

◊ To set your weight goals, go to the "weight-height-body build charts," including the explanation in Chapter 2 in the section "How Much Should I Weigh?" and a chart in the back of the book. For insight into how to reach those goals—in terms of many calories you can consume and how much exercise you'll need—refer to Chapter 2 entitled "My 'Calorie Allowance' for Losing Weight."

◊ Keep those scales handy. Step on the scales every single day and weigh.

◊ Get on with your program! And good luck!

Epilogue

Family and the Lifetime Commitment to Weight Control

Anita Smith

In the previous chapters, you have traveled with Dr. David Bell as he recalled his decades of being overweight. You also have traveled with him as he described his joy in launching a successful battle in 2003 to lose that weight and, for four years now, to keep the weight off.

As the medical writer who has worked with Dr. Bell on this book, I have been struck by the strong commitment Dr. Bell feels to keeping his weight under control for the rest of his life.

There is no doubt in my mind that Dr. Bell's commitment is driven partly out of his desire to stay healthy and active as long as possible so he can enjoy his family to the fullest.

Dr. Bell is very aware that his family members have worried through the years about his being overweight. He also is aware that his family members are both proud and relieved that he has lost the weight.

As Dr. Bell came toward the end of this book's chapters, he and I discussed how strongly family dynamics enter into the weight issue. He commented that many of you who need to lose substantial amounts of weight also have family members who worry about you—family members who also will be your best cheerleaders if you lose that weight.

We felt it could be constructive to share with you some individual personal perspectives from Dr. Bell's family members—perspectives about how they view Dr. Bell's weight-loss journey (and how long it took him to make up his mind to make that journey). We decided to collect these individual perspectives from Dr. Bell's mother, wife, and three sons.

In so doing, we hope that members of Dr. Bell's own family will share some insights that will strike home with you and with your family members. Perhaps you or your family members will see yourselves in some of these Bell family perspectives. Perhaps for readers of this book some of these Bell family insights will help to spur forward some of your own successful weight-loss stories.

A Mother's Perspective

Violet "Vi" Bell remembered her eldest son's weight being an issue from the time he came into the world.

"Of our three children, David was by far the biggest baby at birth—over 10 pounds," she said in an interview several months before her death in July 2007. "As a child David always ate more and was heavier than his younger brother and sister. In addition to eating a lot, I think David also ate the wrong things, particularly breads."

Vi Bell said it's easy to see why her son liked bread so much, since the delicious bread in Ireland can be very tempting. "Oh, I think in Ireland bread can be *anybody's* downfall," said Vi Bell, at the time 87 and still making her home in a suburb of Belfast, the Northern Ireland city where she and her late husband lived much of their married lives and reared their children. "Here in Ireland we still have all these good breads, and we also have such a great selection of breads."

For Vi, seeing her eldest son trim and fit in his early 60s was a gift. "Throughout his life, until recently, David was almost always too fat," she said. "Now he looks great!" When she first learned that her physician son was on a serious program to lose weight and keep it off, she was delighted. "It was so wonderful to hear that and then to see him looking so good!" she said.

During the years when David was growing up, the issue of how to deal with David's overweight condition produced different viewpoints from his parents. On the one hand, his mother was inclined to encourage her son to eat healthier foods and smaller portions and to get off some of the weight. However, her husband, James, took a different slant on the situation. He didn't want Vi to harass their eldest about his weight.

"My husband told me, 'Now, don't keep at David about his weight,'" said Vi. "He particularly thought it was a dreadful thing for me to say anything to David about what he was eating while the family was at the table enjoying a meal. My husband just wanted the food to be served and for everyone to be happy while they were eating it!"

This whole issue of food and extra pounds was something that Vi and James Bell actually had experienced differently themselves. Vi could identify with what it was like to have to watch one's weight. She herself tended to carry a few pounds more than the "charts" would have considered ideal, even though she was nowhere close to having the kind of weight problem son David was developing. "Now, I was not what you would call 'fat,' but I was a bit round," she said. As for her husband, being overweight was far from being an issue with him. After son David had grown from an overweight child into an overweight adult, David would reflect that he certainly didn't take after his dad's side of the family when it came to the weight issue. "My father was always thin, thin!" said David Bell. "In fact, my father's whole side of the family was a rather gaunt, skinny group. While I would describe my father as being thin, I would describe my father's older brother as being *very* thin!"

Despite the differences in views between David's mom and dad as to how to manage his weight, David's mom recalled that at some point when he was still a young boy a decision was made to take David to a dietitian, to obtain some advice about dieting. In one sense, the advice the Bells received from the dietitian worked; for David did lose weight. In another sense, it didn't work; because David gained back the weight, very quickly. "After we went to see that dietitian, David actually in about five weeks time lost a stone of weight (Great Britain unit equal to about 14 pounds). But then he gained it all back," said Vi.

The mother said one of the things that pleased her most about David's current weight loss was that this time the solution seems to be a long-term one. At the time she shared her perspective for this book, Vi had seen her son in recent weeks when he and wife Jocelyn made a trip to Ireland, to visit relatives and attend a family wedding. Some two years had passed since Vi had first seen David all slimmed down as a result of his one-meal-a-day and one-hour-of-exercise-a-day program. On his more recent visit to Ireland he was still slim, perhaps even a bit thinner than she had last seen him. "Isn't it wonderful that this time when David got this weight off, he has kept it off!" she said.

When Vi actually talked to son David directly about what she thought about his losing from around 325 pounds down to 210, she told him simply, "David, now your weight suits you."

A Wife Becomes a Weight-Loss Advocate

Almost from the time Jocelyn Johnston married David Bell, Jocelyn became involved in her husband's diets—his efforts to get a few pounds off here and there.

Since Jocelyn was working as a registered nurse and a registered nurse-midwife in the early years of their marriage, she was keenly aware of the health hazards of her husband's overweight condition. She encouraged him to lose weight, and she willingly helped with the diets. In fact, she *encouraged* the diets.

"We would try this diet and then that diet," said Jocelyn. "One of the earlier diets I remember was when I was pregnant with our first child, son James, who was born two years after we married. I remember this diet particularly because it required that David start off the day by eating a full breakfast. Oh, I well remember being pregnant and cooking those breakfast meals for David early in the morning and feeling so ill!"

As he went from one diet to another through the years, David Bell would lose some weight on a diet and regain that weight, and then lose some weight on the next diet and regain that weight, and on and on.

Then came the time in recent years when Jocelyn's husband more or less *stopped losing* any weight; all he did was *gain* weight.

"I became very concerned about David's health, because he just kept putting on weight and then more weight. Always before he would get to a certain point with his weight, and then he would go on a diet and lose some. But the time came when there was no break to lose any weight at all. No matter what I said, David just kept piling the weight on. He was getting so heavy that to me it seemed like he just didn't care. It appeared that David really was trying to buck the system medically. David felt that it was fine for him to tell his patients to keep their weight under control for health reasons, but at the same time David's words about weight and health didn't apply to David."

Jocelyn said that when mealtime rolled around in the Bell household, her husband would eat and eat and then eat some more.

"It was as though David felt that if there was *any* food on the table, in any shape or form, that food had to be eaten. And *he* was the one who would eat it. I would give him one helping. And no matter what size a helping that was, if there was more in the pot he would eat that, too."

At the same time Dr. David Bell was getting heavier and heavier, he also was not under the care of a personal physician and was not getting regular checkups.

Jocelyn Johnston Bell couldn't get her own health-related training, knowledge and experience out of her head. As one who for years had been a practicing nurse and nurse-midwife, she knew her severely overweight husband could be sitting on a bad-health time bomb.

"I often would ask David if he didn't think he needed to see a physician, if he didn't need to get a doctor besides himself to look after him, instead of just self-diagnosing. But, just as he did about his eating, he ignored my advice. He just kept going the way he was going."

All in all, Jocelyn said she felt her husband was conveying a message that he wanted to be left alone about his weight and his healthcare, that what he did in regard to those issues was his own business. "I felt that David's attitude was, 'Well, it's *my* life,' " said Jocelyn.

As part of his career as a physician specializing in diabetes and metabolism within a university academic health sciences center, Dr. Bell traveled a great deal to give medical lectures, in cities and towns around the nation and also abroad.

When he was away on his travels, Jocelyn worried about him even more. She knew he was burning the candle at both ends—working long hours, overeating, not getting enough rest. Her anxiety level often was quite high when he was out of town.

"I had this fear that while David was traveling he would suffer a heart attack or a stroke, like in his hotel room or whatever. For some reason, my biggest fear for him was specifically a heart attack. Generally when David is traveling he telephones me every night. But on occasion if he gets back to the hotel real late, or if he falls asleep, I don't hear from him. Back in those days when he was so overweight and working so hard, when he was out of town I really worried if the phone didn't ring when I thought it should at night. Until I would hear his voice on the phone, there were times I would think, 'Is David out there somewhere dead?' "

By mid-2003, Jocelyn had stepped up her pressure on her husband to at least avail himself of some basic health screening tests—to find out where he stood in regard to his cholesterol, blood pressure, and blood sugar.

"I was *really* on his case to have these tests," she said.

So, one night when Dr. Bell was attending the American Diabetes Association meeting in New Orleans, Louisiana, he telephoned Jocelyn to tell her that he had finally taken her advice and had gotten those tests earlier that day.

"In that phone conversation, David started out by telling me that he had gotten these tests at the booths in the Exhibit Hall there, where they were having the diabetes meeting."

As it turned out, he gave his wife the good news first. Then things went downhill from there. This is her recollection:

"David started off the conversation by telling me, 'I had my cholesterol checked today. And it was normal.' Well, I sat there thinking, 'Now, I can't believe that one!' And I couldn't. I just could not believe the way David was eating and gaining all that weight that he really had normal-level cholesterol. Actually, I'll have to say that in a sense I felt kind of disgusted when he told he that he had this normal cholesterol reading. I thought, 'If David is overeating and gaining all this weight and still he has normal cholesterol, how am I ever going to convince him that he needs to be on a diet and get this weight under control? He will see no need to change.' "

And then, in this memorable phone conversation, David Bell dropped the bombshell on his wife. He told her that he also had gotten his blood pressure checked that day. And, quite unlike his normal cholesterol reading, the blood pressure reading was far, far *above* normal levels. In fact, his blood pressure reading was so off the charts that he could easily suffer a stroke or a heart attack at any minute. He explained that he had gone straight to a local drugstore and gotten medications to start bringing down the blood pressure.

"I could tell during that conversation that David was really very worried about his blood pressure, as anybody would be with blood pressure that high. I was very, very concerned," said Jocelyn. "It was worrisome to me that David wasn't actually checking himself into a hospital immediately."

But Jocelyn said she also felt that if her husband did indeed survive this crisis period, things were about to change for the better—not because of anything she said to him, but because of what he already knew himself. "From the time I received that phone call, I felt that David was making a decision to change, that he had realized he couldn't just keep going the way he was going."

From the time he arrived back home, Jocelyn knew she had correctly sensed her husband's frame of mind. "Even though for so long David had not listened about overeating and gaining all this weight, it became apparent that he had become so concerned about this blood pressure, and also that he knew one way to help himself was to lose weight."

Jocelyn believed that her husband would indeed lose weight now that he had made up his mind to do so. "I know that once David sets his mind to accomplishing something, he is very focused," she said.

Even knowing that, Jocelyn still was impressed with the ease and consistency with which Dr. Bell proceeded and stuck with his rather unusual diet and exercise plan.

"Once he settled on this one meal a day and one hour of exercise a day, it really didn't even appear to be that difficult for him," she said. "The weight just began coming off. And, as you can see, the weight is still off. I really don't think he will regain it."

All along the way, she said she has seen one bonus after another that her husband has received.

"One thing is how well his clothes fit and how he seems to feel now about clothes. David is so tall and he was so overweight that for so long it was a real problem for him to get clothes to fit properly. He had to have everything made. And he didn't seem to care particularly about clothes. Now for the first time I see David really getting excited about having new clothes. Although he still has some things made, he also now is able to buy at least some things in stores. And he really looks so good in his clothes! When a person is thinner, clothes just tend to fit better."

Some of the bonuses of his weight loss are for both Jocelyn and David.

"Before David's weight loss, he did all this loud snoring and also had sleep apnea, where he would stop breathing," she said. "Why, with the sleep apnea there were times when I would think, 'It seems so long since David even took a breath!' I would have to kick him or punch him to get him started breathing again. Since his weight loss, he snores only very occasionally. And there is no sleep apnea. I no longer have to crank him up, to give him a jump-start! *Both* of us sleep better."

And, perhaps above all, as her husband still travels and gives those medical lectures, Jocelyn no longer is on pins and needles waiting for a reassuring phone call that he's all right.

"We all know we have no guarantees in life. But at the same time I know that by losing weight—by eating healthily and exercising regularly—David has lowered his health risks tremendously. Now that he's thin and looks and seems so healthy, his traveling for me is not nearly as stressful."

When Jocelyn talks about her husband's weight-loss—and about how he was finally frightened into that weight-loss program because of his blood pressure reading—she remembers a statement he made to her.

She smiles the knowing smile of a wife who had long worried about her husband's weight and who had tried in vain to get him to take the weight off. "You know what David said when he called from New Orleans to tell me that one of those health screening tests had shown he had a real problem—that he had this terrible high blood pressure? He said, 'Jocelyn, the only reason I took these tests was to prove to you that I *did not* have any health problems, that nothing was wrong with me.' "

Eldest Son Follows in his Father's Footsteps

David and Jocelyn Bell have three children, all sons. The eldest of the three is James, the namesake of his paternal grandfather. Numerous times during James's 34 years, he has heard people comment on the striking similarities between himself and his father.

"Actually, I've been told I'm the son who is *most* like my father," said James.

He himself acknowledges the similarities. He looks a lot like his dad; he talks and moves a lot like him. As a physician, his dad for decades worked killer hours. As an Indianapolis, Indiana, attorney (a litigator specializing in white-collar criminal defense), James admits he quickly became a committed workaholic.

Also, James picked up some of his dad's bad habits when it came to eating too much food and getting too little exercise, and gaining weight—a good 20 to 30 pounds overweight. At a young age, James also began paying the price health-wise. Like his dad, James was diagnosed with high blood pressure (at age 30)—not nearly as high as his dad's blood pressure, but high enough to require medication. James also had very high cholesterol.

As of this writing, James's weight is down to normal, his exercise is up, and his cholesterol and blood pressure are under control. (In addition to diet and exercise, he still takes medication to control the blood pressure.)

James said his dad's success with his weight-loss program has been a great example for him to follow. He reflects on the health habits of himself and his father yesterday and today.

"When I was growing up, I came to know that an evening of fun for my father was to sit down and talk with friends or family members and have a few drinks and eat some food, a lot of food. I remember as a kid going to Ireland with my parents, and I can recall how much fried food the Irish people ate. I can remember some Irish people referring to what they called 'a good fry.' Now, sometimes they were referring to what they were having for breakfast! They would fry up everything—from eggs to bacon to bread. I mean, they even had fried bread. And, being the good Irishman that he is, my dad loved all that food—sitting around eating it while he visited with people he enjoyed."

As James went through college and then on to his career in law, his own idea of socializing was much like his father's. When he took time to relax, he usually did it with food and drink. Like his dad, he was eating a lot of food. Like his dad, James was eating too much food, too many helpings, and too much dessert. James also signed up for the fast-food habit that is embraced by much of American society.

"Like my father, my idea of having a good time was to sit down and talk with my friends. While I was doing that, I'd have a few beers with maybe a pizza or some burgers or chicken wings!" said James. "There were times at lunch when I would have two cheeseburgers, a large order of French fries, and a large Coke. Later, when I went on Weight-Watchers, I learned that in one meal I was using up all the food-unit allowances for an entire day!"

James got by pretty well weight-wise when he was in college, likely due to the fact he was a competitive swimmer and thus was burning calories through hours of swimming each day.

"After I stopped swimming competitively, and after I became an attorney and started working so many hours, I found it hard to fit exercise into my schedule and I didn't make exercise a priority. Actually, I never exercised unless I had an absolutely free day."

With little exercise and a lot of food, James started putting on weight.

Then came the symptoms that were real health problems. James was burning the midnight oil, working very long hours preparing for a big trial and feeling quite stressed. "I was sitting at my desk actually getting short of breath. I mean, I was barely 30 years old. That was scary!" He went to see a physician, and in so doing he learned he had high blood pressure and high cholesterol. He launched a diet and exercise program to address the problems.

As James has gotten his own lifestyle under control health-wise, he has turned for guidance to his own physician in Indianapolis and also to his father. The timing of James's learning about his own health issues came just about the time his own father had addressed his life-threatening health problem and had lost a great deal of weight.

"My father is an excellent physician, a good person with whom I can consult. I find his advice very creditable, very helpful," said James. "Too,

Dad understands where I am coming from with my own health issues—especially the cholesterol and high blood pressure and weight loss. And my father is in a situation to give me advice based on his experience with his own weight loss and healthier lifestyle."

James personally observed some of his dad's experiences as Dr. Bell transformed himself from being one who was doing it the wrong way to being one who is doing it the right way.

For example, the eldest Bell son can recall seeing firsthand some times when his dad made it clear that he felt the rules didn't apply to him.

"When I was a college student in Indiana I sometimes would go to medical meetings with my father—meetings at which Dad would be speaking," said James. "I can recall an occasion sitting down to a meal with Dad and some of his colleagues after Dad made this medical presentation. And we were sitting there eating this dessert at dinner and this guy said to my dad, 'After what you just told us in your presentation, we really shouldn't be eating this dessert.' And my dad laughed and told him, 'Oh, diets are just for patients!' "

In contrast, James also can recall hearing his dad's chilling description of the day in New Orleans when he found out that the rules did indeed apply to him.

"My dad told me, 'James, I learned that I had 'blow-your-brains-out' blood pressure!' "

Now that he sees his dad singing a far different tune about weight and diet and exercise, James is convinced that his dad is in this good-health program for the long haul.

"I think my dad has really seized the moment and wants to do whatever he can to increase his chances he will have a healthy future for as long as possible," said James.

James said there had been times in his life when he wondered about his dad's feelings about his own mortality. "My grandfather, my dad's father, died of cancer at a young age, at 61. That's younger than my dad is now. There were times when my dad made comments that led me to suspect that perhaps Dad might think that he, too, would die at a young age, just like his father had done. If Dad really did feel that way, I don't think he does anymore. He's still traveling and doing medical lectures. He and my mother are taking trips together. Dad is having a great time, and he continues to keep his weight down."

James said that just as his dad has made some health and lifestyle conversions and changes in the past couple of years, he himself also has made changes. Those changes include more than action-oriented alterations in James' daily habits; the changes also include a new attitude and new point of view as it relates to taking care of himself. James speaks of his discoveries about how important it is that he keep himself as healthy as possible, not only for the sake of himself, but also for his family, including his wife Anne.

"I think my dad and I both have learned some meanings about moderation and balance," said James. "I have learned about moderation and balance at a younger age than Dad and with the help of Dad. But both Dad and I have learned. Through moderation you can enjoy a balance in life. You can still do a great job in your work, and you still can take care of your family, and you still can take time for fun. But at the same time you can focus enough time and effort on taking care of yourself in a balanced way—by eating and drinking in moderation, exercising regularly, and getting good healthcare. That all adds up to using some moderation in order to get that balance you need."

Middle Son Lends Dad Some Advice

Of the three Bell sons, the only one living near Dr. David Bell when he carried out his weight-loss program was middle son Michael. At age 31, Michael lives with his wife Laura in a Birmingham, Alabama, neighborhood not far from his parents. His job is in the loan department of a Birmingham bank. And one of his pastimes is exercise and physical activity. In college Michael played ice hockey and soccer; today he still works out regularly at a gym and keeps himself in shape.

As a part of the exercise component of his father's weight-loss program, it was Michael who advised his dad about how to work with weights and gave his father a starter set of weights as a gift. This all came about after David Bell was deep into his dieting and exercise and felt he needed some upper-body toning. Longtime physician Dr. Bell, who traditionally had been the one in the Bell family handing out advice to other people, went to his middle son seeking some advice about weight-lifting exercise. Michael was glad to be consulted and prompt to help. "I just showed Dad a few basics with the weights. I don't want him to hurt himself," said Michael.

As is true with other Bell family members, Michael was very relieved when his father decided to lose weight and followed through with it. Back in the days when his father was working such long hours and was so terribly overweight, Michael actually shared his mother's worry that his dad would die suddenly while on one of his medical-lecture trips. Although he didn't share his fears with his mom, it turned out that mother and son were thinking similar dismal thoughts. "I just felt that Dad couldn't last forever going like that and being so overweight," said Michael. "When he was away traveling, I never knew when the telephone call would come from someone saying it was over for him."

Through the years, it sometimes was difficult for Michael to understand how his dad could be a widely acclaimed expert in metabolism and diabetes but at the same time not practice what he preached.

"I always thought it was ironic that my dad was a well-respected doctor who would talk to patients about controlling their eating habits, and that people would listen to him, even though he wasn't following his own advice as a doctor," said Michael. "I mean, my dad had all this knowledge about nutrition and weight control, and yet he was not using that knowledge to help himself."

It is Michael's opinion that one of the problems during those years was that Dr. Bell invested most all his attention on others and virtually none on himself. "Dad loves his family and of course wants to make sure they are okay, and he has always loved his patients and has devoted much attention to them," said Michael. "I really believe that Dad was just trying so hard to help everybody else that he wasn't thinking about himself and was not helping himself with his own health problems."

Michael said he has been impressed that once his dad made the decision to lose the weight and keep it off, he had been committed to carrying out his diet and exercise program. The middle son said he admires his father for that stickability. He said that on previous occasions he already had seen that stickability trait in his father. "Oh, Dad is like that when he makes up his mind! Back when he decided to give up pipe-smoking, he did not do it gradually; he just decided one day to give up the pipe, and he stuck with it. The same thing has been true with his diet and exercise and losing the weight. I really respect that. You know, Dad has done something that is so hard for many people who need to lose weight. People can do short-term thinking about weight loss and say, 'I can wait till tomorrow to start losing weight.' But then their waiting can turn into never doing it. I'm glad my dad did it."

The Changing Views of the Youngest Son

When the Bells' youngest son, Andrew, was growing up, he just felt that his dad's large body size went along with the "big" image he had of his dad in general.

His dad was very tall—6 feet, 5 inches. His dad also was quite heavy.

At the same time, his dad's accomplishments as an endocrinologist were quite expansive. He was revered as a superb clinician, an excellent manager of care for patients with diabetes and other metabolic conditions. He was heavily into research and teaching. Seeds were being planted in his career that would make him more and more in demand as a speaker on the medical-lecture circuit, nationally and internationally.

Andrew recalled that from his view his dad just cut such a big presence when he walked into a room. Since Andrew was so proud of his father, everything about him seemed BIG and it all fit together.

"I thought my dad was larger than life anyhow," said Andrew. "So in a way I saw his size with a 'well, my dad is bigger than your dad' view! Dad's being so big in a way was kind of fun to me back when I was a kid."

As Andrew got a little older, his view of his dad's overweight state began to change a bit. "I began to realize the possible health consequences of Dad's size. And it was worrisome to me."

Gradually Andrew began to spot some things about his dad that made him feel the same way his two older brothers felt; Andrew came to believe that his dad was focused so much on other people that he wasn't taking care of himself.

For Andrew, and for his brothers as well, some of that insight came from working temporary part-time jobs in their dad's academic-health-sciences-center medical practice.

"At one time or another, my two brothers and I all worked some for my dad at the clinic. In doing that, we really realized how much he did for his patients," said Andrew. He said his dad's tremendous dedication to patients at work and then to family at home left him little time for himself. (Ironically, a stint that Andrew had as a teenager working for his overweight dad involved doing some clerical work for Dr. Bell's research project about patients' weight-loss!)

At age 27, bachelor Andrew Bell now lives in Indianapolis, Indiana, where he is regional automobile loan specialist for a Minneapolis, Minnesota-based bank.

Since Andrew and his older brother James both live in Indiana and their parents live hundreds of miles away in Alabama, weeks and sometimes months go by between visits. Andrew said the fact he wasn't seeing his dad frequently made his dad's weight-loss and body-toning appearance changes all that more noticeable.

"Why, once Dad started losing this weight, every time I would see him he had lost more weight, and it was making pretty dramatic changes," said Andrew. "By the time he got down to his ideal weight, it was pretty mind-blowing to me! You know, when Dad learned that he had this severe high blood pressure problem, I really do think it just about scared the life out of him. Just think of how much healthier it has to be for him now than at the weight back when he was so big. I mean, I will tell you that I think my dad's weight loss is great—really great!"

Dr. Bell: For Himself, and for Others

For Dr. David Bell, there are increasing incentives to keep his weight off—to keep eating healthily and to keep exercising.

He's very to-the-point about his growing incentives for being into weight-control for the long haul, for a lifetime:

"I intend to keep this weight off for myself. I feel so much better, and my chances of living a healthier, longer life are so much better," said Dr. Bell.

"Too, I plan to keep the weight off for my family. I wouldn't want to let them down.

"And then there's still another incentive, a new added incentive, isn't there? I mean, if I were to write this book encouraging readers to lose weight and keep it off, and then if I were to fall off the wagon myself and start regaining my weight, well I would really have egg on my face, wouldn't I?"

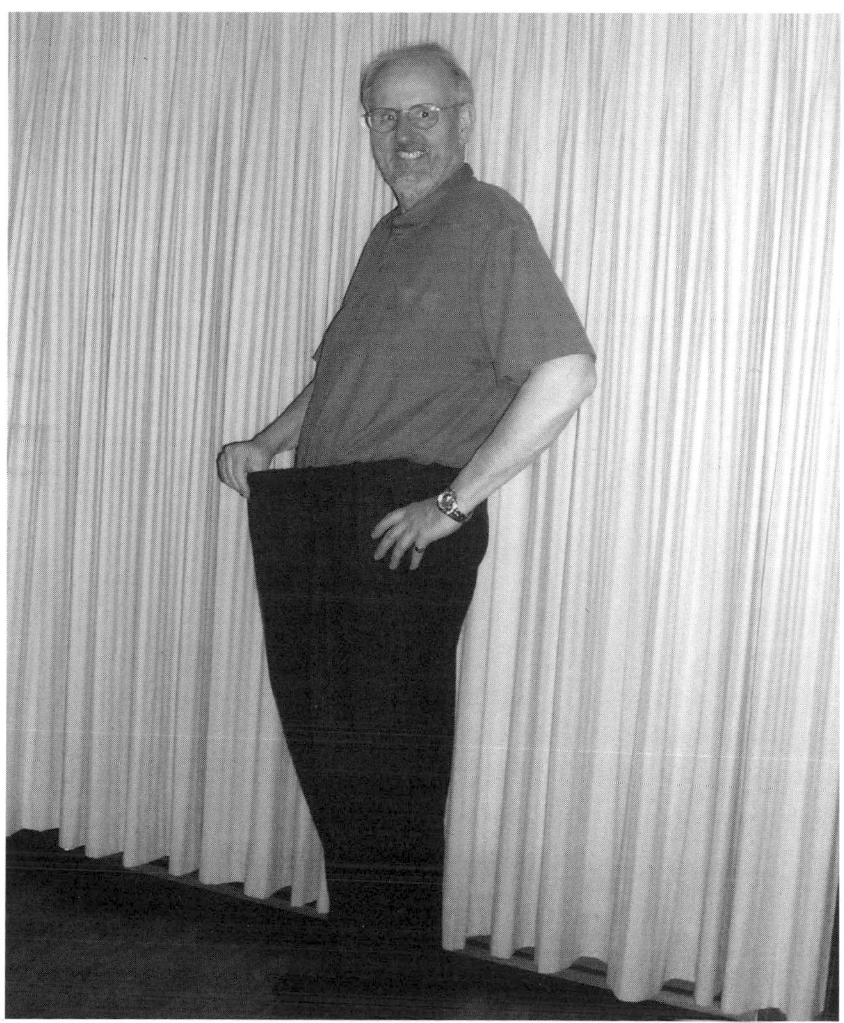

"How good it is!" In December 2004, I had fun trying on a pair of pants I wore prior to my dramatic weight loss.

IDEAL WEIGHT LEVELS

Per Height/Bone Structure (danger levels in parentheses)

	Height	Small	Medium	Large
Women	5'0"	90 (108)	100 (120)	110 (132)
	5'1"	95 (114)	105 (126)	116 (140)
	5'2"	99 (120)	110 (132)	121 (145)
	5'3"	104 (125)	115 (138)	126 (152)
	5'4"	108 (130)	120 (144)	132 (158)
	5'5"	113 (135)	125 (150)	138 (166)
	5'6"	117 (141)	130 (156)	143 (171)
	5'7"	122 (146)	135 (161)	148 (176)
	5'8"	126 (150)	140 (168)	154 (184)
	5'9"	131 (157)	145 (174)	159 (192)
	5'10"	135 (162)	150 (180)	165 (198)
	5'11"	141 (169)	155 (186)	170 (204)
	6'0"	146 (176)	160 (192)	176 (212)
Men	5'0"	96 (115)	106 (127)	117 (140)
	5'1"	101 (121)	112 (136)	123 (147)
	5'2"	106 (127)	118 (142)	130 (156)
	5'3"	112 (133)	124 (149)	136 (163)
	5'4"	117 (141)	130 (156)	143 (172)
	5'5"	122 (146)	136 (163)	149 (179)
	5'6"	128 (154)	142 (170)	156 (187)
	5'7"	133 (160)	148 (178)	162 (196)
	5'8"	139 (167)	154 (185)	170 (204)
	5'9"	144 (173)	160 (192)	176 (211)
	5'10"	149 (179)	166 (199)	183 (220)
	5'11"	155 (188)	172 (206)	189 (227)
	6'0"	160 (192)	178 (214)	196 (235)
	6'1"	166 (199)	184 (221)	202 (242)
	6'2"	171 (205)	190 (228)	209 (251)
	6'3"	176 (211)	196 (235)	215 (259)
	6'4"	182 (218)	202 (242)	222 (266)
	6'5"	185 (222)	206 (247)	226 (271)

Index

Q

R

S

T

U

V

W